CLINICAL COMPANION
FOR
PSYCHIATRIC–MENTAL
HEALTH NURSING

CLINICAL COMPANION FOR PSYCHIATRIC–MENTAL HEALTH NURSING

Karen Lee Fontaine, RN, MSN, AASECT
Professor, Purdue University Calumet
Hammond, Indiana

Carol Ren Kneisl, RN, MS, APRN, DABFN
President and Director of Continuing Education,
Nursing Transitions
Clinical and Legal Consultant, Orange Beach, Alabama

Eileen Trigoboff, RN, APRN/PHM–BC, DNS, DABFN
Private Practice Clinical Nurse Specialist, Psychiatry
Clinical and Legal Consultant
Office of Mental Health in New York State
Buffalo, New York

PEARSON
Prentice
Hall

Upper Saddle River, New Jersey 07458

Library of Congress Catalogin-in-Publication Data
Fontaine, Karen Lee, (date)
  Clinical companion for psychiatric–mental health nursing/Karen Lee Fontaine, Carol Ren Kneisl, Eileen Trigoboff.
    p. ; cm.
Includes bibliographical references and index.
  ISBN 0-13-098241-5 (alk. paper)
  1. Psychiatric nursing.
  [DNLM: 1. Psychiatric Nursing. 2. Mental Disorders—nursing. WY 160 F678c 2004] I. Kneisl, Carol Ren. II. Trigoboff, Eileen. III. Title.
  RC440 .F54 2004
  610.73'68--dc21

                                                                    2003002303

Pearson Education LTD., *London*
Pearson Education Australia PTY, Limited, *Sydney*
Pearson Education Singapore, Pte. Ltd
Pearson Education North Asia Ltd, *Hong Kong*
Pearson Education Canada, Ltd., *Toronto*
Pearson Educatión de Mexico, S.A. de C.V.
Pearson Education—Japan, *Tokyo*
Pearson Education Malaysia, Pte. Ltd
Pearson Education, Upper Saddle River, New Jersey

10 9 8 7 6 5 4 3 2 1
ISBN 0-13-098241-5

CONTENTS

PREFACE

The *Clinical Companion for Psychiatric–Mental Health Nursing* is a convenient reference when caring for clients in various clinical settings. It can be used as a supplement to a variety of mental health nursing texts. The compact design of the *Clinical Companion* makes it easy to take to clinical settings. It provides essential information in an easy-to-read format and provides a bridge for nursing students between the classroom and the clinical situation. Professional nurses new to mental health nursing will find that this text is a good overview of skills to be developed in this area of practice. Experienced mental health nurses will find this text a quick refresher of their knowledge base.

ORGANIZATION

The *Clinical Companion* provides a quick reference for standards of practice, diagnostic studies, DSM-IV-TR diagnoses, legal issues, and standard precautions. The nursing process section reviews assessment, North American Nursing Diagnosis Association (NANDA) diagnoses, and planning through using Nursing Outcome Classifications. Implementation is based on Nursing Intervention Classifications. Psychoeducation is stressed as a critical part of nursing intervention, as knowledge empowers people to make informed decisions regarding their health status, plan for maintaining wellness, and illness care choices. Various types of therapies are highlighted under nursing interventions. Psychotropic medications are presented clearly and concisely to provide the student with a quick reference while in the clinical setting.

Client–nurse experiences come to life in the Clinical Applications section, which covers 24 of the most common problematic behaviors. These behaviors appear in alphabetical order for easy access. Each behavior adheres to the following format:

- Basic definition
- Assessment cues
- Interventions and rationales

- Client illustration, featuring a statement by the client followed by two possible responses on the part of the nurse. Rationales for each response are included.

The last step of the nursing process, evaluation and documentation, and practice-based research conclude the *Clinical Companion*. A bibliography and an index are found in the back of the book.

ACKNOWLEDGMENTS

Our thanks to the editorial staff at Prentice Hall, especially Elisabeth Garofalo and Maura Connor, for their guidance and support. We thank all of our students over the years, whose questions stimulated us, and whose understandings broadened our knowledge base.

REVIEWERS

Rebecca Crews Gruener, MS
Associate Professor
Louisiana State University at Alexandria
Alexandria, Louisiana

Kathleen Rose-Grippa, PhD, RN
School of Nursing
Ohio University
Athens, Ohio

Maryellen McBride, MN, ARNP, CARN
Assistant Professor
Washburn University
Topeka, Kansas

Joan Wilk, PhD, RN
Associate Professor
University of Wisconsin-Milwaukee
Kenosha, Wisconsin

CLINICAL COMPANION
FOR
PSYCHIATRIC–MENTAL
HEALTH NURSING

QUICK REFERENCE

STANDARDS OF PRACTICE

In the 2000 *Scope and Standards of Psychiatric–Mental Health Nursing Practice,* the American Nurses' Association (ANA) delineates the standards to which nurses are held, both legally and ethically.*

Standard I. Assessment: The psychiatric–mental health nurse collects patient health data.

Rationale: The assessment interview, which requires linguistically and culturally effective communication skills, interviewing, behavioral observation, record reviews, and comprehensive assessment of the patient and relevant systems, enables the psychiatric–mental health nurse to make sound clinical judgments and plan appropriate interventions with the patient.

Standard II. Diagnosis: The psychiatric–mental health nurse analyzes the assessment data in determining diagnoses.

Rationale: The basis for providing psychiatric–mental health nursing care is the recognition and identification of patterns of response to actual or potential psychiatric illnesses, mental health problems, and potential comorbid physical illnesses.

Standard III. Outcome Identification: The psychiatric–mental health nurse identifies expected outcomes individualized to the patient.

Rationale: Within the context of providing nursing care, the ultimate goal is to influence mental health outcomes and improve the patient's health status.

Standard IV. Planning: The psychiatric–mental health nurse develops a plan of care that is negotiated among the patient, nurse, family, and health care team and prescribes evidence-based interventions to attain expected outcomes.

Rationale: A plan of care is used to guide therapeutic interventions systematically, document progress, and achieve the expected patient outcomes.

---

*Reprinted with permission from the American Nurses Association, American Psychiatric Nurses Association, International Society of Psychiatric–Mental Health Nurses, *Scope and Standards of Psychiatric–Mental Health Nursing Practice*, © 2000 American Nurses Foundation/American Nurses Association, Washington, DC.

Standard V. Implementation: The psychiatric–mental health nurse implements the interventions identified in the plan of care.

Rationale: In implementing the plan of care, psychiatric–mental health nurses use a wide range of interventions designed to prevent mental and physical illness, and promote, maintain, and restore mental and physical health. Psychiatric–mental health nurses select interventions according to their level of practice. At the basic level, nurses may select counseling, milieu therapy, promotion of self-care activities, intake screening and evaluation, psychobiological interventions, health teaching, case management, health promotion and health maintenance, crisis intervention, community-based care, psychiatric home health care, telehealth, and a variety of other approaches to meet the mental health needs of patients. In addition to the intervention options available to the basic-level psychiatric–mental health nurse, at the advanced level the Advanced Practice Registered Nurse–Psychiatric Mental Health (APRN–PMH) may provide consultation, engage in psychotherapy, and prescribe pharmacological agents in accordance with state statutes or regulations.

Standard Va. Counseling: The psychiatric–mental health nurse uses counseling interventions to assist patients in improving or regaining their previous coping abilities, fostering mental health, and preventing mental illness and disability.

Standard Vb. Milieu Therapy: The psychiatric–mental health nurse provides, structures, and maintains a therapeutic environment in collaboration with the patient and other health care clinicians.

Standard Vc. Promotion of Self-Care Activities: The psychiatric–mental health nurse structures interventions around the patient's activities of daily living to foster self-care and mental and physical well-being.

Standard Vd. Psychobiological Interventions: The psychiatric–mental health nurse uses knowledge of psychobiological interventions and applies clinical skills to restore the patient's health and prevent further disability.

Standard Ve. Health Teaching: The psychiatric–mental health nurse, through health teaching, assists patients in achieving satisfying, productive, and healthy patterns of living.

Standard Vf. Case Management: The psychiatric–mental health nurse provides case management to coordinate comprehensive health services and to ensure continuity of care.

Standard Vg. Health Promotion and Health Maintenance: The psychiatric–mental health nurse employs strategies and interventions to promote and maintain health and prevent mental illness.

Advance Practice Interventions Vh–Vj

Standard Vh. Psychotherapy

Standard Vi. Prescriptive Authority and Treatment

Standard Vj. Consultation

Standard VI. Evaluation: The psychiatric–mental health nurse evaluates the patient's progress in attaining expected outcomes.

Rationale: Nursing care is a dynamic process involving change in the patient's health status over time, giving rise to the need for data, different diagnoses, and modification in the plan of care. Therefore, evaluation is a continuous process of appraising the effect of nursing and the treatment regimen on the patient's health status and expected outcomes.

COMMON DIAGNOSTIC STUDIES

MRI

Magnetic resonance imaging (MRI) produces high quality images of the inside of the human body. It gives us a look into bodily structures and the problems within those structures. MRI began as a tomographic imaging technique similar to CT scans that produced an image of the nuclear magnetic resonance (NMR) signal in a thin section through the human body. MRI has advanced beyond a tomographic imaging technique to a volume imaging technique that can provide us with a two- or three-dimensional representation of any very small point in the body. It has a variety of uses that include diagnosis and evaluating treatment.

MRI is often used to diagnose the specific nature of an internal physical problem. Clients undergoing an MRI can choose how the test will be performed. Traditional MRI machines have a restricted space within which the client must remain immobile. Newer MRI machines provide a greater sense of comfort to the client through a larger, more open, or less constrictive testing area. This has made it possible for clients to feel more comfortable when undergoing this necessary diagnostic procedure.

SPECT

A single-photon emission computed tomography (SPECT) brain scan is a diagnostic nuclear medicine imaging procedure that permits visualization of brain function by obtaining three-dimensional images of the brain. SPECT brain scans can show areas of the brain and how well the various regions of the brain are functioning. The SPECT camera takes a series of pictures that shows how efficiently blood flows through the brain.

PET

Positron emission tomography scans (PET) imaging has been in clinical use since the early 1990s, while its history dates back to early research in the 1950s. PET differs from anatomic-based imaging modalities in that it assesses the level of metabolic activity and perfusion in various organ systems and provides measurements of how the body functions in processes such as perfusion, metabolism, and receptors. The process produces images based on the detection of gamma rays that are emitted by a radioactive substance tagged to a natural body compound, commonly glucose.

In neurology, PET scans of the brain are used to evaluate people who have memory disorders of undetermined etiology, brain tumors, or seizure disorders unresponsive to therapy, and are therefore candidates for surgery. PET is also used in Alzheimer's disease therapy to monitor outcomes with a variety of newer medications. In psychiatry, PET has shown that successful treatment of obsessive-compulsive disorder (OCD) with medication or with behavior therapy produces similar reductions in activity in the brain's basal ganglia. The scan also shows that OCD involves a specific biological abnormality.

A fairly new clinical use for PET scans is treatment responsiveness. PET imaging after certain kinds of therapy (such as chemotherapy) can be predictive of a clinical response and nonresponse. This would affect morbidity, increase the quality of life, and avoid the costs of ineffective therapy.

There is a new hybrid CT/PET scanning process that offers exquisite images fusing metabolism with anatomic landmarks.

MMPI-2

The Minnesota Multiphasic Personality Inventory-2 (MMPI-2) is an objective personality test for the assessment of psychopathology in adults. It is a paper and pencil test (which can also be administered on a computer or presented orally) designed to assess a number of major patterns of personality, emotional, and behavioral disorders. There are 567 statements that the client marks true or false. The MMPI takes between 40 and 90 minutes to complete and is scored by a psychologist.

The score obtained for this test gives an overall profile of the individual's emotional, psychological, and interpersonal functioning from which important information about the psychiatric diagnosis can be obtained. Specific areas of functioning, which can be revealed by the test results, include problems with hypochondriasis, depression, hysteria, psychopathy, paranoia, anxiety, thought disorder, and mania.

BECK DEPRESSION INVENTORY

The Beck Depression Inventory II is a 21-item self-report instrument developed in 1961 to screen for depressive symptoms and their severity in people 13 years of age and older. Answers are based on events of the past two weeks. It takes about 10 minutes to complete. Each item is rated from 0 to 3. High score is 63.

The scores indicate the presence and level of depression:

- 0–13 indicates minimal depression.
- 14–19 indicates mild.
- 20–28 indicates moderate.
- 29–63 indicates severe depression.

CAGE

The CAGE is most frequently used for the detection of alcoholism in clinical settings. It is part of a thorough, nonjudgmental substance use assessment and consists of interview questions likely to elicit accurate answers regarding problems with alcohol. CAGE is a mnemonic for these four questions:

1. Have you ever felt like you should **C**ut down on your drinking?
2. Have people **A**nnoyed you by criticizing your drinking?
3. Have you ever felt bad or **G**uilty about your drinking?
4. Have you ever had a drink in the morning as an **E**ye-opener to get rid of a hangover?

Positive answers to two or more of these four questions suggest concerns about alcohol use.

AIMS

The Abnormal Involuntary Movement Scale (AIMS) is one of the tools used to detect tardive dyskinesia (TD), a side effect of many psychotropic medications. TD is characterized by arrhythmic, involuntary movements that can include lip smacking, tongue protrusion, rocking, foot tapping, pelvic thrusts, finger movements, and grimace-like facial expressions. The AIMS examination procedure includes a review of the muscles of the

- Face
- Jaw
- Tongue
- Extremities
- Trunk

for abnormal, involuntary movements occurring in an irregular pattern and formalized on a numbered scale from absent (0) to severe (4) movements. Scoring depends on whether the movement occurs spontaneously or must be activated, and the highest severity observed earns the score for that area of the body.

Primary prevention of TD is accomplished by careful initial assessment of a client's needs, as well as continual evaluation during the course of pharmacologic treatment. Regular assessment is required to detect the presence of TD and to determine the level of severity. Careful documentation of regular assessments with the AIMS will reveal the presence or worsening of TD.

DSM-IV-TR DIAGNOSES

Mental disorders are classified in the *Diagnostic and Statistical Manual of Mental Disorders,* Fourth Edition, Text Revision (DSM-IV-TR), published by the American Psychiatric Association. All members of the health care team use the DSM-IV-TR, which groups client information into five categories, called axes. Axis I includes a majority of the mental disorders. Axis II lists long-lasting problems, including personality disorders and developmental disorders. Both Axis I and Axis II describe the intrapersonal area of functioning. Axis III describes the physical problems of disorders that must be considered when planning the client's treatment program. If there are no physical problems, the diagnosis on Axis III will be stated as "none." Axis IV describes the psychosocial stressors (acute and long lasting) occurring in the past year that have contributed to the current mental disorder. Nurses should be aware of how many stressors have occurred and how much change each stressor caused in the life of the client. Axis V rates the highest level of psychological, social, and occupational functioning the client has achieved in the past year, as well as the current level of functioning. It is especially important to be sensitive to cultural differences and expectations when rating clients on Axis V.

DSM-IV-TR CLASSIFICATION*

NOS = Not Otherwise Specified

An *x* appearing in a diagnostic code indicates that a specific code number is required.

An ellipsis (. . .) is used in the names of certain disorders to indicate that the name of a specific mental disorder or general medical condition should be inserted when recording the name (e.g., 293.0 Delirium Due to Hypothyroidism).

If criteria are currently met, one of the following severity specifiers may be noted after the diagnosis:

Mild
Moderate
Severe

If criteria are no longer met, one of the following specifiers may be noted:

In Partial Remission
In Full Remission
Prior History

*Reprinted with permission from the *Diagnostic and Statistical Manual of Mental Disorders,* Fourth Edition, Text Revision Copyright 2000, American Psychiatric Association.

Disorders Usually First Diagnosed in Infancy, Childhood, or Adolescence

MENTAL RETARDATION

Note: These are coded on Axis II.

317	Mild Mental Retardation
318.0	Moderate Mental Retardation
318.1	Severe Mental Retardation
318.2	Profound Mental Retardation
319	Mental Retardation, Severity Unspecified

LEARNING DISORDERS

315.00	Reading Disorder
315.1	Mathematics Disorder
315.2	Disorder of Written Expression
315.9	Learning Disorder NOS

MOTOR SKILLS DISORDER

315.4	Developmental Coordination Disorder

COMMUNICATION DISORDERS

315.31	Expressive Language Disorder
315.32	Mixed Receptive-Expressive Language Disorder
315.39	Phonological Disorder
307.0	Stuttering
307.9	Communication Disorder NOS

PERVASIVE DEVELOPMENTAL DISORDERS

299.00	Autistic Disorder
299.80	Rett's Disorder
299.10	Childhood Disintegrative Disorder
299.80	Asperger's Disorder
299.80	Pervasive Developmental Disorder NOS

ATTENTION-DEFICIT AND DISRUPTIVE BEHAVIOR DISORDERS

314.xx	Attention-Deficit/Hyperactivity Disorder
.01	Combined Type
.00	Predominantly Inattentive Type
.01	Predominantly Hyperactive-Impulsive Type
314.9	Attention-Deficit/Hyperactivity Disorder NOS
312.xx	Conduct Disorder
.81	Childhood-Onset Type
.82	Adolescent-Onset Type
.89	Unspecified Onset
313.81	Oppositional Defiant Disorder
312.9	Disruptive Behavior Disorder NOS

FEEDING AND EATING DISORDERS OF INFANCY OR EARLY CHILDHOOD

307.52	Pica
307.53	Rumination Disorder
307.59	Feeding Disorder of Infancy or Early Childhood

Tic Disorders

307.23 Tourette's Disorder
307.22 Chronic Motor or Vocal Tic Disorder
307.21 Transient Tic Disorder
       Specify if: Single Episode/Recurrent
307.20 Tic Disorder NOS

Elimination Disorders

___.__ Encopresis
787.6 With Constipation and Overflow Incontinence
307.7 Without Constipation and Overflow Incontinence
307.6 Enuresis (Not Due to a General Medical Condition)
       Specify type: Nocturnal Only/Diurnal Only/Nocturnal and Diurnal

Other Disorders of Infancy, Childhood, or Adolescence

309.21 Separation Anxiety Disorder
       Specify if: Early Onset
313.23 Selective Mutism
313.89 Reactive Attachment Disorder of Infancy or Early Child-
       hood
       Specify type: Inhibited Type/Disinhibited Type
307.3 Stereotypic Movement Disorder
       Specify if: with Self-Injurious Behavior
313.9 Disorder of Infancy, Childhood, or Adolescence NOS

Delirium, Dementia, and Amnestic and Other Cognitive Disorders

Delirium

293.0 Delirium Due to . . . *[Indicate the General Medical
       Condition]*
___.__ Substance Intoxication Delirium *(refer to Substance-
       Related Disorders for substance-specific codes)*
___.__ Substance Withdrawal Delirium *(refer to Substance-
       Related Disorders for substance-specific codes)*
___.__ Delirium Due to Multiple Etiologies *(code each of the
       specific etiologies)*
780.09 Delirium NOS

Dementia

294.xx[†] Dementia of the Alzheimer's Type. With Early Onset
         (also code 331.0 Alzheimer's disease on Axis III)
    .10 Without Behavioral Disturbance
    .11 With Behavioral Disturbance
294.xx[†] Dementia of the Alzheimer's Type, With Late Onset
         (also code 331.0 Alzheimer's disease on Axis III)
    .10 Without Behavioral Disturbance
    .11 With Behavioral Disturbance
290.xx   Vascular Dementia

[†]ICD-9-CM code valid after October 1, 2000.

.40   Uncomplicated
.41   With Delirium
.42   With Delusions
.43   With Depressed Mood
        Specify if: With Behavioral Disturbance

Code presence or absence of a behavioral disturbance in the fifth digit for Dementia Due to a General Medical Condition:

        0 = Without Behavioral Disturbance
        1 = With Behavioral Disturbance

294.1x[†]   Dementia Due to HIV Disease *(also code 042 HIV on Axis III)*

294.1x[†]   Dementia Due to Head Trauma *(also code 854.00 head injury on Axis III)*

294.1x[†]   Dementia Due to Parkinson's Disease *(also code 332.0 Parkinson's disease on Axis III)*

294.1x[†]   Dementia Due to Huntington's Disease *(also code 333.4 Huntington's disease on Axis III)*

294.1x[†]   Dementia Due to Pick's Disease *(also code 331.1 Pick's disease on Axis III)*

294.1x[†]   Dementia Due to Creutzfeldt-Jakob Disease *(also code 046.1 Creutzfeldt-Jakob disease on Axis III)*

294.1x[†]   Dementia Due to . . . *[Indicate the General Medical Condition not listed above] (also code the general medical condition on Axis III)*

___.___   Substance-Induced Persisting Dementia *(refer to Substance-Related Disorders for substance-specific codes)*

___.___   Dementia Due to Multiple Etiologies *(code each of the specific etiologies)*

294.8   Dementia NOS

Amnestic Disorders

294.0   Amnestic Disorder Due to . . . *[Indicate the General Medical Condition]*
          Specify if: Transient/Chronic

___.___   Substance-Induced Persisting Amnestic Disorder *(refer to Substance-Related Disorders for substance-specific codes)*

294.8   Amnestic Disorder NOS

Other Cognitive Disorders

294.9   Cognitive Disorder NOS

Mental Disorders Due to a General Medical Condition Not Elsewhere Classified

293.89   Catatonic Disorder Due to . . . *[Indicate the General Medical Condition]*

310.1   Personality Change Due to . . . *[Indicate the General Medical Condition]*

Specify type: Labile Type/Disinhibited Type/Aggressive Type/Apathetic Type/Paranoid Type/Other Type/Combined Type/Unspecified Type

293.9 Mental Disorder NOS Due to . . . *[Indicate the General Medical Condition]*

Substance-Related Disorders

The following specifiers apply to Substance Dependence as noted:

[a]With Physiological Dependence/Without Physiological Dependence
[b]Early Full Remission/Early Partial Remission/Sustained Full Remission/ Sustained Partial Remission
[c]In a Controlled Environment
[d]On Agonist Therapy

The following specifiers apply to Substance-Induced Disorders as noted:

[I]With Onset During Intoxication/[W]With Onset During Withdrawal

ALCOHOL-RELATED DISORDERS
Alcohol Use Disorders

303.90	Alcohol Dependence[a,b,c]
305.00	Alcohol Abuse

Alcohol-Induced Disorders

303.00	Alcohol Intoxication
291.81	Alcohol Withdrawal
	Specify if: With Perceptual Disturbances
291.0	Alcohol Intoxication Delirium
291.0	Alcohol Withdrawal Delirium
291.2	Alcohol-Induced Persisting Dementia
291.1	Alcohol-Induced Persisting Amnestic Disorder
291.x	Alcohol-Induced Psychotic Disorder
.5	With Delusions[I,W]
.3	With Hallucinations[I,W]
291.89	Alcohol-Induced Mood Disorder[I,W]
291.89	Alcohol-Induced Anxiety Disorder[I,W]
291.89	Alcohol-Induced Sexual Dysfunction[I]
291.89	Alcohol-Induced Sleep Disorder[I,W]
291.9	Alcohol-Related Disorder NOS

AMPHETAMINE (OR AMPHETAMINE-LIKE)-RELATED DISORDERS
Amphetamine Use Disorders

304.40	Amphetamine Dependence[a,b,c]
305.70	Amphetamine Abuse

Amphetamine-Induced Disorders

292.89	Amphetamine Intoxication
	Specify if: With Perceptual Disturbances
292.0	Amphetamine Withdrawal

292.81   Amphetamine Intoxication Delirium
292.xx   Amphetamine-Induced Psychotic Disorder
  .11   With Delusions[I]
  .12   With Hallucinations[I]
292.84   Amphetamine-Induced Mood Disorder[I,W]
292.89   Amphetamine-Induced Anxiety Disorder[I]
292.89   Amphetamine-Induced Sexual Dysfunction[I]
292.89   Amphetamine-Induced Sleep Disorder[I,W]
292.9   Amphetamine-Related Disorder NOS

CAFFEINE-RELATED DISORDERS
Caffeine-Induced Disorders
305.90   Caffeine Intoxication
292.89   Caffeine-Induced Anxiety Disorder[I]
292.89   Caffeine-Induced Sleep Disorder[I]
292.9   Caffeine-Related Disorder NOS

CANNABIS-RELATED DISORDERS
Cannabis Use Disorders
304.30   Cannabis Dependence[a,b,c]
305.20   Cannabis Abuse

Cannabis-Induced Disorders
292.89   Cannabis Intoxication
         Specify if: With Perceptual Disturbance
292.81   Cannabis Intoxication Delirium
292.xx   Cannabis-Induced Psychotic Disorder
  .11   With Delusions[I]
  .12   With Hallucinations[I]
292.89   Cannabis-Induced Anxiety Disorder[I]
292.9   Cannabis-Related Disorder NOS

COCAINE-RELATED DISORDERS
Cocaine Use Disorders
304.20   Cocaine Dependence[a,b,c]
305.60   Cocaine Abuse

Cocaine-Induced Disorders
292.89   Cocaine Intoxication
         Specify if: With Perceptual Disturbances
292.0   Cocaine Withdrawal
292.81   Cocaine Intoxication Delirium
292.xx   Cocaine-Induced Psychotic Disorder
  .11   With Delusions[I]
  .12   With Hallucinations[I]
292.84   Cocaine-Induced Mood Disorder[I,W]
292.89   Cocaine-Induced Anxiety Disorder[I,W]
292.89   Cocaine-Induced Sexual Dysfunction[I]
292.89   Cocaine-Induced Sleep Disorder[I,W]
292.9   Cocaine-Related Disorder NOS

HALLUCINOGEN-RELATED DISORDERS
Hallucinogen Use Disorders
304.50   Hallucinogen Dependence[b,c]
305.30   Hallucinogen Abuse

Hallucinogen-Induced Disorders
292.89   Hallucinogen Intoxication
292.89   Hallucinogen Persisting Perception Disorder (Flashbacks)
292.81   Hallucinogen Intoxication Delirium
292.xx   Hallucinogen-Induced Psychotic Disorder
  .11   With Delusions[I]
  .12   With Hallucinations[I]
292.84   Hallucinogen-Induced Mood Disorder[I]
292.89   Hallucinogen-Induced Anxiety Disorder[I]
292.9   Hallucinogen-Related Disorder NOS

INHALANT-RELATED DISORDERS
Inhalant Use Disorders
304.60   Inhalant Dependence[b,c]
305.90   Inhalant Abuse

Inhalant-Induced Disorders
292.89   Inhalant Intoxication
292.81   Inhalant Intoxication Delirium
292.82   Inhalant-Induced Persisting Dementia
292.xx   Inhalant-Induced Psychotic Disorder
  .11   With Delusions[I]
  .12   With Hallucinations[I]
292.84   Inhalant-Induced Mood Disorder[I]
292.89   Inhalant-Induced Anxiety Disorder[I]
292.9   Inhalant-Related Disorder NOS

NICOTINE-RELATED DISORDERS
Nicotine Use Disorder
305.1   Nicotine Dependence[a,b]

Nicotine-Induced Disorders
292.0   Nicotine Withdrawal
292.9   Nicotine-Related Disorder NOS

OPIOID-RELATED DISORDERS
Opioid Use Disorders
304.00   Opioid Dependence[a,b,c,d]
305.50   Opioid Abuse

Opioid-Induced Disorders
292.89   Opioid Intoxication
          Specify if: With Perceptual Disturbances
292.0   Opioid Withdrawal
292.81   Opioid Intoxication Delirium
292.xx   Opioid-Induced Psychotic Disorder
  .11   With Delusions[I]
  .12   With Hallucinations[I]

292.84	Opioid-Induced Mood Disorder[I]
292.89	Opioid-Induced Sexual Dysfunction[I]
292.89	Opioid-Induced Sleep Disorder[I,W]
292.9	Opioid-Related Disorder NOS

PHENCYCLIDINE (OR PHENCYCLIDINE-LIKE)-RELATED DISORDERS
Phencyclidine Use Disorders

| 304.60 | Phencyclidine Dependence[b,c] |
| 305.90 | Phencyclidine Abuse |

Phencyclidine-Induced Disorders

292.89	Phencyclidine Intoxication
	Specify if: With Perceptual Disturbances
292.81	Phencyclidine Intoxication Delirium
292.xx	Phencyclidine-Induced Psychotic Disorder
.11	With Delusions[I]
.12	With Hallucinations[I]
292.84	Phencyclidine-Induced Mood Disorder[I]
292.89	Phencyclidine-Induced Anxiety Disorder[I]
292.9	Phencyclidine-Related Disorder NOS

SEDATIVE-, HYPNOTIC-, OR ANXIOLYTIC-RELATED DISORDERS
Sedative, Hypnotic, or Anxiolytic Use Disorders

| 304.10 | Sedative, Hypnotic, or Anxiolytic Dependence[a,b,c] |
| 305.40 | Sedative, Hypnotic, or Anxiolytic Abuse |

Sedative-, Hypnotic-, or Anxiolytic-Induced Disorders

292.89	Sedative, Hypnotic, or Anxiolytic Intoxication
292.0	Sedative, Hypnotic, or Anxiolytic Withdrawal
	Specify if: With Perceptual Disturbances
292.81	Sedative, Hypnotic, or Anxiolytic Intoxication Delirium
292.81	Sedative, Hypnotic, or Anxiolytic Withdrawal Delirium
292.82	Sedative, Hypnotic, or Anxiolytic-Induced Persisting Dementia
292.83	Sedative-, Hypnotic-, or Anxiolytic-Induced Persisting Amnestic Disorder
292.xx	Sedative-, Hypnotic-, or Anxiolytic-Induced Psychotic Disorder
.11	With Delusions[I,W]
.12	With Hallucinations[I,W]
292.84	Sedative-, Hypnotic-, or Anxiolytic-Induced Mood Disorder[I,W]
292.89	Sedative-, Hypnotic-, or Anxiolytic-Induced Anxiety Disorder[W]
292.89	Sedative-, Hypnotic-, or Anxiolytic-Induced Sexual Dysfunction[I]
292.89	Sedative-, Hypnotic, or Anxiolytic-Induced Sleep Disorder[I,W]
292.9	Sedative-, Hypnotic-, or Anxiolytic-Related Disorder NOS

POLYSUBSTANCE-RELATED DISORDER
304.80   Polysubstance Dependence[a,b,c,d]

OTHER (OR UNKNOWN) SUBSTANCE-RELATED DISORDERS
Other (or Unknown) Substance Use Disorders
304.90   Other (or Unknown) Substance Dependence[a,b,c,d]
305.90   Other (or Unknown) Substance Abuse

Other (or Unknown) Substance-Induced Disorders
292.89   Other (or Unknown) Substance Intoxication
         Specify if: With Perceptual Disturbances
292.0   Other (or Unknown) Substance Withdrawal
         Specify if: With Perceptual Disturbances
292.81   Other (or Unknown) Substance-Induced Delirium
292.82   Other (or Unknown) Substance-Induced Persisting
         Dementia
292.83   Other (or Unknown) Substance-Induced Persisting
         Amnestic Disorder
292.xx   Other (or Unknown) Substance-Induced Psychotic
         Disorder
   .11   With Delusions[I,W]
   .12   With Hallucinations[I,W]
292.84   Other (or Unknown) Substance-Induced Mood
         Disorder[I,W]
292.89   Other (or Unknown) Substance-Induced Anxiety
         Disorder[I,W]
292.89   Other (or Unknown) Substance-Induced Sexual
         Dysfunction[I]
292.89   Other (or Unknown) Substance-Induced Sleep
         Disorder[I,W]
292.9   Other (or Unknown) Substance-Related Disorder NOS

POLYSUBSTANCE-RELATED DISORDER
304.80   Polysubstance Dependence[a,b,c,d]

OTHER (OR UNKNOWN) SUBSTANCE-RELATED DISORDERS
Other (or Unknown) Substance Use Disorders
304.90   Other (or Unknown) Substance Dependence[a,b,c,d]
305.90   Other (or Unknown) Substance Abuse

Other (or Unknown) Substance-Induced Disorders
292.89   Other (or Unknown) Substance Intoxication
         Specify if: With Perceptual Disturbances
292.0   Other (or Unknown) Substance Withdrawal
         Specify if: With Perceptual Disturbances
292.81   Other (or Unknown) Substance-Induced Delirium
292.82   Other (or Unknown) Substance-Induced Persisting
         Dementia
292.83   Other (or Unknown) Substance-Induced Persisting
         Amnestic Disorder

292.xx	Other (or Unknown) Substance-Induced Psychotic Disorder
.11	With Delusions[I,W]
.12	With Hallucinations[I,W]
292.84	Other (or Unknown) Substance-Induced Mood Disorder[I,W]
292.89	Other (or Unknown) Substance-Induced Anxiety Disorder[I,W]
292.89	Other (or Unknown) Substance-Induced Sexual Dysfunction[I]
292.89	Other (or Unknown) Substance-Induced Sleep Disorder[I,W]
292.9	Other (or Unknown) Substance-Related Disorder NOS

Schizophrenia and Other Psychotic Disorders

295.xx   Schizophrenia

The following Classification of Longitudinal Course applies to all subtypes of Schizophrenia:

> Episodic With Interepisode Residual Symptoms (*Specify if:* With Prominent Negative Symptoms)/Episodic With No Interepisode Residual Symptoms
> Continuous (*Specify if:* With Prominent Negative Symptoms)
> Single Episode in Partial Remission (*Specify if:* With Prominent Negative Symptoms)/Single Episode in Full Remission
> Other or Unspecified Pattern

.30	Paranoid Type
.10	Disorganized Type
.20	Catatonic Type
.90	Undifferentiated Type
.60	Residual Type
295.40	Schizophreniform Disorder
	Specify if: Without Good Prognostic Features/With Good Prognostic Features
295.70	Schizoaffective Disorder
	Specify type: Bipolar Type/Depressive Type
297.1	Delusional Disorder
	Specify type: Erotomanic Type/Grandiose Type/Jealous Type/Persecutory Type/Somatic Type/Mixed Type/Unspecified Type
298.8	Brief Psychotic Disorder
	Specify if: With Marked Stressor(s)/Without Marked Stressor(s)/With Postpartum Onset
297.3	Shared Psychotic Disorder
293.xx	Psychotic Disorder Due to . . . *[Indicate the General Medical Condition]*
.81	With Delusions
.82	With Hallucinations
___.__	Substance-Induced Psychotic Disorder *(refer to Substance-Related Disorders for substance-specific codes)*

Specify if: With Onset During Intoxication/With Onset During Withdrawal

298.9 Psychotic Disorder NOS

Mood Disorders

Code current state of Major Depressive Disorder or Bipolar I Disorder in fifth digit:

   1 = Mild
   2 = Moderate
   3 = Severe Without Psychotic Features
   4 = Severe With Psychotic Features
       Specify: Mood-Congruent Psychotic Features/Mood-Incongruent Psychotic Features
   5 = In Partial Remission
   6 = In Full Remission
   0 = Unspecified

The following specifiers apply (for current or most recent episode) to Mood Disorders as noted:

[a]Severity/Psychotic/Remission Specifiers/[b]Chronic/[c]With Catatonic Features/[d]With Melancholic Features/[e]With Atypical Features/[f]With Postpartum Onset

The following specifiers apply to Mood Disorders as noted:

[g]With or Without Full Interepisode Recovery/[h]With Seasonal Pattern/[i]With Rapid Cycling

DEPRESSIVE DISORDERS

296.xx	Major Depressive Disorder	
.2x	Single Episode[a,b,c,d,e,f]	
.3x	Recurrent[a,b,c,d,e,f,g,h]	
300.4	Dysthymic Disorder	

Specify if: Early Onset/Late Onset
Specify if: With Atypical Features

311 Depressive Disorder NOS

BIPOLAR DISORDERS

296.xx	Bipolar I Disorder	
.0x	Single Manic Episode[a,c,f]	

Specify if: Mixed

.40	Most Recent Episode Hypomanic[g,h,i]	
.4x	Most Recent Episode Manic[a,c,f,g,h,i]	
.6x	Most Recent Episode Mixed[a,c,f,g,h,i]	
.5x	Most Recent Episode Depressed[a,b,c,d,e,f,g,h,i]	
.7	Most Recent Episode Unspecified[g,h,i]	
296.89	Bipolar II Disorder[a,b,c,d,e,f,g,h,i]	

Specify (current or most recent episode): Hypomanic/Depressed

301.13	Cyclothymic Disorder
296.80	Bipolar Disorder NOS

293.83   Mood Disorder Due to . . . *[Indicate the General Med-*
          ical Condition]
          Specify type: With Depressive Features/With Major Depressive-
          Like Episode/With Manic Features/With Mixed Features

___.___   Substance-Induced Mood Disorder *(refer to Substance-*
          Related Disorders for substance-specific codes)
          Specify type: With Depressive Features/With Manic
          Features/With Mixed Features
          Specify if: With Onset During Intoxication/With Onset During
          Withdrawal

296.90   Mood Disorder NOS

Anxiety Disorders

300.01   Panic Disorder Without Agoraphobia
300.21   Panic Disorder With Agoraphobia
300.22   Agoraphobia Without History of Panic Disorder
300.29   Specific Phobia
          Specify type: Animal Type/Natural Environment Type/Blood-
          Injection-Injury Type/Situational Type/Other Type
300.23   Social Phobia
          Specify if: Generalized
300.3   Obsessive-Compulsive Disorder
          Specify if: With Poor Insight
309.81   Posttraumatic Stress Disorder
          Specify if: Acute/Chronic
          Specify if: With Delayed Onset
308.3   Acute Stress Disorder
300.02   Generalized Anxiety Disorder
293.84   Anxiety Disorder Due to . . . *[Indicate the General Med-*
          ical Condition]
          Specify if: With Generalized Anxiety/With Panic Attacks/With
          Obsessive-Compulsive Symptoms

___.___   Substance-Induced Anxiety Disorder *(refer to Sub-*
          stance-Related Disorders for substance-specific codes)
          Specify if: With Generalized Anxiety/With Panic Attacks/With
          Obsessive Compulsive Symptoms/With Phobic Symptoms
          Specify if: With Onset During Intoxication/With Onset During
          Withdrawal

300.00   Anxiety Disorder NOS

Somatoform Disorders

300.81   Somatization Disorder
300.82   Undifferentiated Somatoform Disorder
300.11   Conversion Disorder

Specify type: With Motor Symptom or Deficit/With Sensory
Symptom or Deficit/With Seizures or Convulsions/With Mixed
Presentation

307.xx	Pain Disorder
.80	Associated With Psychological Factors
.89	Associated With Both Psychological Factors and a General Medical Condition

Specify if: Acute/Chronic

300.7	Hypochondriasis

Specify if: With Poor Insight

300.7	Body Dysmorphic Disorder
300.82	Somatoform Disorder NOS

Factitious Disorders

300.xx	Factitious Disorder
.16	With Predominantly Psychological Signs and Symptoms
.19	With Predominantly Physical Signs and Symptoms
.19	With Combined Psychological and Physical Signs and Symptoms
300.19	Factitious Disorder NOS

Dissociative Disorders

300.12	Dissociative Amnesia
300.13	Dissociative Fugue
300.14	Dissociative Identity Disorder
300.6	Depersonalization Disorder
300.15	Dissociative Disorder NOS

Sexual and Gender Identity Disorders

SEXUAL DYSFUNCTIONS
The following specifiers apply to all primary Sexual Dysfunctions:

Lifelong Type/Acquired Type
Generalized Type/Situational Type
Due to Psychological Factors/Due to Combined Factors

SEXUAL DESIRE DISORDERS

302.71	Hypoactive Sexual Desire Disorder
302.79	Sexual Aversion Disorder

SEXUAL AROUSAL DISORDERS

302.72	Female Sexual Arousal Disorder
302.72	Male Erectile Disorder

ORGASMIC DISORDERS

302.73	Female Orgasmic Disorder
302.74	Male Orgasmic Disorder
302.75	Premature Ejaculation

SEXUAL PAIN DISORDERS
302.76   Dyspareunia (Not Due to a General Medical Condition)
306.51   Vaginismus (Not Due to a General Medical Condition)

SEXUAL DYSFUNCTION DUE TO A GENERAL MEDICAL CONDITION
625.8   Female Hypoactive Sexual Desire Disorder Due to . . . *[Indicate the General Medical Condition]*
608.89   Male Hypoactive Sexual Desire Disorder Due to . . . *[Indicate the General Medical Condition]*
607.84   Male Erectile Disorder Due to . . . *[Indicate the General Medical Condition]*
625.0   Female Dyspareunia Due to . . . *[Indicate the General Medical Condition]*
608.89   Male Dyspareunia Due to . . . *[Indicate the General Medical Condition]*
625.8   Other Female Sexual Dysfunction Due to . . . *[Indicate the General Medical Condition]*
608.89   Other Male Sexual Dysfunction Due to . . . *[Indicate the General Medical Condition]*
___.__   Substance-Induced Sexual Dysfunction *(refer to Substance-Related Disorders for substance-specific codes)*
         Specify if: With Impaired Desire/With Impaired Arousal/With Impaired Orgasm/With Sexual Pain
         Specify if: With Onset During Intoxication
302.70   Sexual Dysfunction NOS

PARAPHILIAS
302.4   Exhibitionism
302.81   Fetishism
302.89   Frotteurism
302.2   Pedophilia
         Specify if: Sexually Attracted to Males/Sexually Attracted to Females/Sexually Attracted to Both
         Specify if: Limited to Incest
         Specify type: Exclusive Type/Nonexclusive Type
302.83   Sexual Masochism
302.84   Sexual Sadism
302.3   Transvestic Fetishism
         Specify if: With Gender Dysphoria
302.82   Voyeurism
302.9   Paraphilia NOS

GENDER IDENTITY DISORDERS
302.xx   Gender Identity Disorder
   .6   in Children
   .85   in Adolescents or Adults
         Specify if: Sexually Attracted to Males/Sexually Attracted to Females/Sexually Attracted to Both/Sexually Attracted to Neither
302.6   Gender Identity Disorder NOS

302.9   Sexual Disorder NOS

Eating Disorders
307.1   Anorexia Nervosa
          Specify type: Restricting Type: Binge-Eating/Purging Type
307.51   Bulimia Nervosa
          Specify type: Purging Type/Nonpurging Type
307.50   Eating Disorder NOS

Sleep Disorders
PRIMARY SLEEP DISORDERS
Dyssomnias
307.42   Primary Insomnia
307.44   Primary Hypersomnia
          Specify if: Recurrent
347   Narcolepsy
780.59   Breathing-Related Sleep Disorder
307.45   Circadian Rhythm Sleep Disorder
          Specify type: Delayed Sleep Phase Type/Jet Lag Type/Shift
          Work Type/Unspecified Type
307.47   Dyssomnia NOS

Parasomnias
307.47   Nightmare Disorder
307.46   Sleep Terror Disorder
307.46   Sleepwalking Disorder
307.47   Parasomnia NOS

SLEEP DISORDERS RELATED TO ANOTHER MENTAL DISORDER
307.42   Insomnia Related to . . . *[Indicate the Axis I or Axis II*
          Disorder]
307.44   Hypersomnia Related to . . . *[Indicate the Axis I or Axis*
          II Disorder]

OTHER SLEEP DISORDERS
780.xx   Sleep Disorder Due to . . . *[Indicate the General Med-*
          ical Condition]
   .52   Insomnia Type
   .54   Hypersomnia Type
   .59   Parasomnia Type
   .59   Mixed Type
___.__   Substance-Induced Sleep Disorder *(refer to Substance-*
          Related Disorders for substance-specific codes)
          Specify type: Insomnia Type/Hypersomnia Type/Parasomnia
          Type/Mixed Type
          Specify if: With Onset During Intoxication/With Onset During
          Withdrawal

Impulse-Control Disorders Not Elsewhere Classified

312.34	Intermittent Explosive Disorder
312.32	Kleptomania
312.33	Pyromania
312.31	Pathological Gambling
312.39	Trichotillomania
312.30	Impulse-Control Disorder NOS

Adjustment Disorders

309.xx	Adjustment Disorder
.0	With Depressed Mood
.24	With Anxiety
.28	With Mixed Anxiety and Depressed Mood
.3	With Disturbance of Conduct
.4	With Mixed Disturbance of Emotions and Conduct
.9	Unspecified

Specify if: Acute/Chronic

Personality Disorders

Note:*These are coded on Axis II.*

301.0	Paranoid Personality Disorder
301.20	Schizoid Personality Disorder
301.22	Schizotypal Personality Disorder
301.7	Antisocial Personality Disorder
301.83	Borderline Personality Disorder
301.50	Histrionic Personality Disorder
301.81	Narcissistic Personality Disorder
301.82	Avoidant Personality Disorder
301.6	Dependent Personality Disorder
301.4	Obsessive-Compulsive Personality Disorder
301.9	Personality Disorder NOS

Other Conditions That May Be a Focus of Clinical Attention

PSYCHOLOGICAL FACTORS AFFECTING MEDICAL CONDITION

316   . . . *[Specified Psychological Factor] Affecting . . .*
[Indicate the General Medical Condition]
Choose name based on nature of factors:
Mental Disorder Affecting Medical Condition
Psychological Symptoms Affecting Medical Condition
Personality Traits or Coping Style Affecting Medical
   Condition
Maladaptive Health Behaviors Affecting Medical Condi
   tion
Stress-Related Physiological Response Affecting Med
   ical Condition
Other or Unspecified Psychological Factors Affecting
   Medical Condition

MEDICATION-INDUCED MOVEMENT DISORDERS

332.1	Neuroleptic-Induced Parkinsonism
333.92	Neuroleptic Malignant Syndrome
333.7	Neuroleptic-Induced Acute Dystonia
333.99	Neuroleptic-Induced Acute Akathisia
333.82	Neuroleptic-Induced Tardive Dyskinesia
333.1	Medication-Induced Postural Tremor
333.90	Medication-Induced Movement Disorder NOS

OTHER MEDICATION-INDUCED DISORDER

995.2	Adverse Effects of Medication NOS

RELATIONAL PROBLEMS

V61.9	Relational Problem Related to a Mental Disorder or General Medical Condition
V61.20	Parent-Child Relational Problem
V61.10	Partner Relational Problem
V61.8	Sibling Relational Problem
V62.81	Relational Problem NOS

PROBLEMS RELATED TO ABUSE OR NEGLECT

V61.21	Physical Abuse of Child
	(code 995.54 if focus of attention is on victim)
V61.21	Sexual Abuse of Child
	(code 995.53 if focus of attention is on victim)
V61.21	Neglect of Child
	(code 995.52 if focus of attention is on victim)
___.__	Physical Abuse of Adult
V61.12	(if by partner)
V62.83	(if by person other than partner)
	(code 995.81 if focus of attention is on victim)
___.__	Sexual Abuse of Adult
V61.12	(if by partner)
V62.83	(if by person other than partner)
	(code 995.83 if focus of attention is on victim)

ADDITIONAL CONDITIONS THAT MAY BE A FOCUS OF CLINICAL ATTENTION

V15.81	Noncompliance With Treatment
V65.2	Malingering
V71.01	Adult Antisocial Behavior
V71.02	Child or Adolescent Antisocial Behavior
V62.89	Borderline Intellectual Functioning
	Note: *This is coded on Axis II.*
780.9	Age-Related Cognitive Decline
V62.82	Bereavement
V62.3	Academic Problem
V62.2	Occupational Problem
313.82	Identity Problem
V62.89	Religious or Spiritual Problem

| V62.4 | Acculturation Problem |
| V62.89 | Phase of Life Problem |

Additional Codes

300.9	Unspecified Mental Disorder (nonpsychotic)
V71.09	No Diagnosis or Condition on Axis I
799.9	Diagnosis or Condition Deferred on Axis I
V71.09	No Diagnosis on Axis II
799.9	Diagnosis Deferred on Axis II

Multiaxial System

Axis I	Clinical Disorders
	Other Conditions That May Be a Focus of Clinical Attention
Axis II	Personality Disorders
	Mental Retardation
Axis III	General Medical Conditions
Axis IV	Psychosocial and Environmental Problems
Axis V	Global Assessment of Functioning

MULTIAXIAL ASSESSMENT

A multiaxial system involves an assessment on several axes, each of which refers to a different domain of information that may help the clinician plan treatment and predict outcome. There are five axes included in the DSM-IV multiaxial classification:

Axis I	Clinical Disorders
	Other Conditions That May Be a Focus of Clinical Attention
Axis II	Personality Disorders
	Mental Retardation
Axis III	General Medical Conditions
Axis IV	Psychosocial and Environmental Problems
Axis V	Global Assessment of Functioning

The use of the multiaxial system facilitates comprehensive and systematic evaluation with attention to the various mental disorders and general medical conditions, psychosocial and environmental problems, and level of functioning that might be overlooked if the focus were on assessing a single presenting problem. A multiaxial system provides a convenient format for organizing and communicating clinical information, for capturing the complexity of clinical situations, and for describing the heterogeneity of individuals presenting with the same diagnosis. In addition, the multiaxial system promotes the application of the biopsychosocial model in clinical, educational, and research settings.

The rest of this section provides a description of each of the DSM-IV axes. In some settings or situations, clinicians may prefer not to use the multiaxial system. For this reason, guidelines for reporting the results of a DSM-IV assessment without applying the formal multiaxial system are provided at the end of this section.

AXIS I: CLINICAL DISORDERS—OTHER CONDITIONS THAT MAY BE A FOCUS OF CLINICAL ATTENTION

Axis I is for reporting all the various disorders or conditions in the Classification except for the Personality Disorders and Mental Retardation (which are reported on Axis II). The major groups of disorders to be reported on Axis I are listed in the box below. Also reported on Axis I are Other Conditions That May Be a Focus of Clinical Attention.

When an individual has more than one Axis I disorder, all of these should be reported. If more than one Axis I disorder is present, the principal diagnosis or the reason for visit should be indicated by listing it first. When an individual has both an Axis I and an Axis II disorder, the principal diagnosis or the reason for visit

---

AXIS I

Clinical Disorders

Other Conditions That May Be a Focus of Clinical Attention

Disorders Usually First Diagnosed in Infancy, Childhood, or Adolescence (*excluding Mental Retardation, which is diagnosed on Axis II*)

Delirium, Dementia, and Amnestic and Other Cognitive Disorders

Mental Disorders Due to a General Medical Condition

Substance-Related Disorders

Schizophrenia and Other Psychotic Disorders

Mood Disorders

Anxiety Disorders

Somatoform Disorders

Factitious Disorders

Dissociative Disorders

Sexual and Gender Identity Disorders

Eating Disorders

Sleep Disorders

Impulse-Control Disorders Not Elsewhere Classified

Adjustment Disorders

Other Conditions That May Be a Focus of Clinical Attention

will be assumed to be on Axis I unless the Axis II diagnosis is followed by the qualifying phrase "(Principal Diagnosis)" or "(Reason for Visit)." If no Axis I disorder is present, this should be coded as V71.09. If an Axis I diagnosis is deferred, pending the gathering of additional information, this should be coded as 799.9.

AXIS II: PERSONALITY DISORDERS AND MENTAL RETARDATION

Axis II is for reporting Personality Disorders and Mental Retardation. It may also be used for noting prominent maladaptive personality features and defense mechanisms. The listing of Personality Disorders and Mental Retardation on a separate axis ensures that consideration will be given to the possible presence of Personality Disorders and Mental Retardation that might otherwise be overlooked when attention is directed to the usually more florid Axis I disorders. The coding of Personality Disorders on Axis II should not be taken to imply that their pathogenesis or range of appropriate treatment is fundamentally different from that for the disorders coded on Axis I. The disorders to be reported on Axis II are listed in the box below.

In the common situation in which an individual has more than one Axis II diagnosis, all should be reported. When an individual has both an Axis I and an Axis II diagnosis and the Axis II diagnosis is the principal diagnosis or the reason for visit, this should be indicated by adding the qualifying phrase "(Principal Diagnosis)" or "(Reason for Visit)" after the Axis II diagnosis. If no Axis II disorder is present, this should be coded as V71.09. If an Axis II diagnosis

---

AXIS II

Personality Disorders

Mental Retardation

Paranoid Personality Disorder	Narcissistic Personality Disorder
Schizoid Personality Disorder	Avoidant Personality Disorder
Schizotypal Personality Disorder	Dependent Personality Disorder
Antisocial Personality Disorder	Obsessive-Compulsive Personality Disorder
Borderline Personality Disorder	Personality Disorder Not Otherwise Specified
Histrionic Personality Disorder	Mental Retardation

is deferred, pending the gathering of additional information, this should be coded as 799.9.

Axis II may also be used to indicate prominent maladaptive personality features that do not meet the threshold for a Personality Disorder (in such instances, no code number should be used). The habitual use of maladaptive defense mechanisms may also be indicated on Axis II.

AXIS III: GENERAL MEDICAL CONDITIONS

Axis III is for reporting current general medical conditions that are potentially relevant to the understanding or management of the individual's mental disorder. These conditions are classified outside the "Mental Disorders" chapter of ICD-9-CM (and outside Chapter V of ICD-10). A listing of the broad categories of general medical conditions is given in the box below.

As discussed in the "Introduction," the multiaxial distinction among Axis I, Axis II, and Axis III disorders does not imply that

AXIS III

General Medical Conditions (with ICD-9-CM codes)

Infectious and Parasitic Diseases (001–139)

Neoplasms (140–239)

Endocrine, Nutritional, and Metabolic Diseases and Immunity Disorders (240–279)

Diseases of the Blood and Blood-Forming Organs (280–289)

Diseases of the Nervous System and Sense Organs (320–389)

Diseases of the Circulatory System (390–459)

Diseases of the Respiratory System (460–519)

Diseases of the Digestive System (520–579)

Diseases of the Genitourinary System (580–629)

Complications of Pregnancy, Childbirth, and the Puerperium (630–676)

Diseases of the Skin and Subcutaneous Tissue (680–709)

Diseases of the Musculoskeletal System and Connective Tissue (710–739)

Congenital Anomalies (740–759)

Certain Conditions Originating in the Perinatal Period (760–779)

Symptoms, Signs, and Ill-Defined Conditions (780–799)

Injury and Poisoning (800–999)

there are fundamental differences in their conceptualization, that mental disorders are unrelated to physical or biological factors or processes, or that general medical conditions are unrelated to behavioral or psychosocial factors or processes. The purpose of distinguishing general medical conditions is to encourage thoroughness in evaluation and to enhance communication among health care providers.

General medical conditions can be related to mental disorders in a variety of ways. In some cases it is clear that the general medical condition is directly etiological to the development or worsening of mental symptoms and that the mechanism for this effect is physiological. When a mental disorder is judged to be a direct physiological consequence of the general medical condition, a Mental Disorder Due to a General Medical Condition should be diagnosed on Axis I and the general medical condition should be recorded on both Axis I and Axis III. For example, when hypothyroidism is a direct cause of depressive symptoms, the designation on Axis I is 293.83 Mood Disorder Due to Hypothyroidism, With Depressive Features, and the hypothyroidism is listed again and coded on Axis III as 244.9.

In those instances in which the etiological relationship between the general medical condition and the mental symptoms is insufficiently clear to warrant an Axis I diagnosis of Mental Disorder Due to a General Medical Condition, the appropriate mental disorder (e.g., Major Depressive Disorder) should be listed and coded on Axis I; the general medical condition should only be coded on Axis III.

There are other situations in which general medical conditions are recorded on Axis III because of their importance to the overall understanding or treatment of the individual with the mental disorder. An Axis I disorder may be a psychological reaction to an Axis III general medical condition (e.g., the development of 309.0 Adjustment Disorder With Depressed Mood as a reaction to the diagnosis of carcinoma of the breast). Some general medical conditions may not be directly related to the mental disorder but nonetheless have important prognostic or treatment implications (e.g., when the diagnosis on Axis I is 296.30 Major Depressive Disorder, Recurrent, and on Axis III is 427.9 arrhythmia, the choice of pharmacotherapy is influenced by the general medical condition; or when a person with diabetes mellitus is admitted to the hospital for an exacerbation of schizophrenia and insulin management must be monitored).

When an individual has more than one clinically relevant Axis III diagnosis, all should be reported. If no Axis III disorder is present, this should be indicated by the notation "Axis III: None." If an Axis III diagnosis is deferred, pending the gathering of additional information, this should be indicated by the notation "Axis III: Deferred."

AXIS IV: PSYCHOSOCIAL AND ENVIRONMENTAL PROBLEMS

Axis IV is for reporting psychosocial and environmental problems that may affect the diagnosis, treatment, and prognosis of mental disorders (Axes I and II). A psychosocial or environmental problem may be a negative life event, an environmental difficulty or deficiency, a familial or other interpersonal stress, an inadequacy of social support or personal resources, or other problem relating to the context in which a person's difficulties have developed. So-called positive stressors, such as job promotion, should be listed only if they constitute or lead to a problem, as when a person has difficulty adapting to the new situation. In addition to playing a role in the initiation or exacerbation of a mental disorder, psychosocial problems may also develop as a consequence of a person's psychopathology or may constitute problems that should be considered in the overall management plan.

When an individual has multiple psychosocial or environmental problems, the clinician may note as many as are judged to be relevant. In general, the clinician should note only those psychosocial and environmental problems that have been present during the year preceding the current evaluation. However, the clinician may choose to note psychosocial and environmental problems occurring prior to the previous year if these clearly contribute to the mental disorder or have become a focus of treatment—for example, previous combat experiences leading to Posttraumatic Stress Disorder.

In practice, most psychosocial and environmental problems will be indicated on Axis IV. However, when a psychosocial or environmental problem is the primary focus of clinical attention, it should also be recorded on Axis I, with a code derived from the section "Other Conditions That May Be a Focus of Clinical Attention."

For convenience, the problems are grouped together in the following categories:

- **Problems with primary support group**—e.g., death of a family member; health problems in family; disruption of family by separation, divorce, or estrangement; removal from the home; remarriage of parent; sexual or physical abuse; parental overprotection; neglect of child; inadequate discipline; discord with siblings; birth of a sibling

- **Problems related to the social environment**—e.g., death or loss of friend; inadequate social support; living alone; difficulty with acculturation; discrimination; adjustment of life-cycle transition (such as retirement)
- **Educational problems**—e.g., illiteracy; academic problems; discord with teachers or classmates; inadequate school environment
- **Occupational problems**—e.g., unemployment; threat of job loss; stressful work schedule; difficult work conditions; job dissatisfaction; job change; discord with boss or co-workers
- **Housing problems**—e.g., homelessness; inadequate housing; unsafe neighborhood; discord with neighbors or landlord
- **Economic problems**—e.g., extreme poverty; inadequate finances; insufficient welfare support
- **Problems with access to health care services**—e.g., inadequate health care services; transportation to health care facilities unavailable; inadequate health insurance
- **Problems related to interaction with the legal system/ crime**—e.g., arrest; incarceration; litigation; victim of crime
- **Other psychosocial and environmental problems**—e.g., exposure to disasters, war, other hostilities; discord with nonfamily caregivers such as counselor, social worker, or physician; unavailability of social service agencies

When using the Multiaxial Evaluation Report Form, the clinician should identify the relevant categories of psychosocial and environmental problems and indicate the specific factors involved. If a recording form with a checklist of problem categories is not used, the clinician may simply list the specific problems on Axis IV.

AXIS V: GLOBAL ASSESSMENT OF FUNCTIONING

Axis V is for reporting the clinician's judgment of the individual's overall level of functioning. This information is useful in planning treatment and measuring its impact, and in predicting outcome.

The reporting of overall functioning on Axis V can be done using the Global Assessment of Functioning (GAF) Scale. The GAF Scale may be particularly useful in tracking the clinical progress of individuals in global terms, using a single measure. The GAF Scale is to be rated with respect only to psychological, social, and occupational functioning. The instructions specify, "Do not include impairment in functioning due to physical (or environmental) limitations."

AXIS IV

Psychosocial and Environmental Problems

Problems with primary support group
Problems related to the social environment
Educational problems
Occupational problems
Housing problems
Economic problems
Problems with access to health care services
Problems related to interaction with the legal system/crime
Other psychosocial and environmental problems

The GAF scale is divided into 10 ranges of functioning. Making a GAF rating involves picking a single value that best reflects the individual's overall level of functioning. The description of each 10-point range in the GAF scale has two components: the first part covers symptom severity, and the second part covers functioning. The GAF rating is within a particular decile if **either** the symptom severity **or** the level of functioning falls within the range. For example, the first part of the range 41–50 describes "serious symptoms (e.g., suicidal ideation, severe obsessional rituals, frequent shoplifting)" and the second part includes "any serious impairment in social, occupational, or school functioning (e.g., no friends, unable to keep a job)." It should be noted that in situations where the individual's symptom severity and level of functioning are discordant, the final GAF rating always reflects the worse of the two. For example, the GAF rating for an individual who is a significant danger to self but is otherwise functioning well would be below 20. Similarly, the GAF rating for an individual with minimal psychological symptomatology but significant impairment in functioning (e.g., an individual whose excessive preoccupation with substance use has resulting in loss of job and friends but no other psychopathology) would be 40 or lower.

In most instances, ratings on the GAF Scale should be for the current period (i.e., the level of functioning at the time of the evaluation) because ratings of current functioning will generally reflect the need for treatment or care. In order to account for day-to-day variability in functioning, the GAF rating for the "current period" is sometimes operationalized as the lowest level of functioning for the past week. In some settings, it may be useful to note the GAF Scale rating both at time of admission and at time of discharge. The GAF Scale may also be rated for other time periods (e.g., the highest level of functioning for at least a few months during the past year). The GAF Scale is reported on Axis V as follows: "GAF =," followed by the GAF rating from 0 to 100, followed by the time period reflected by the rating in parentheses—for example, "(current)," "(highest level in past year)," "(at discharge)."

In order to ensure that no elements of the GAF scale are overlooked when a GAF rating is being made, the following method for determining a GAF rating may be applied:

Step 1: Starting at the top level, evaluate each range by asking "is **either** the individual's symptom severity OR level of functioning worse than what is indicated in the range description?"

Step 2: Keep moving down the scale until the range that best matches the individual's symptom severity OR the level of functioning is reached, **whichever is worse.**

Step 3: Look at the next lower range as a double-check against having stopped prematurely. This range should be too severe on **both** symptom severity **and** level of functioning. If it is, the appropriate range has been reached (continue with step 4). If not, go back to step 2 and continue moving down the scale.

Step 4: To determine the specific GAF rating within the selected 10-point range, consider whether the individual is functioning at the higher or lower end of the 10-point range. For example, consider an individual who hears voices that do not influence his behavior (e.g., someone with long-standing schizophrenia who accepts his hallucinations as part of his illness). If the voices occur relatively infrequently (once a week or less), a rating of 39 or 40 might be most appropriate. In contrast, if the individual hears voices almost continuously, a rating of 31 or 32 would be more appropriate.

In some settings, it may be useful to assess social and occupational disability and to track progress in rehabilitation independent of the severity of the psychological symptoms.

Global Assessment of Functioning (GAF) Scale

Consider psychological, social, and occupational functioning on a hypothetical continuum of mental health-illness. Do not include impairment in functioning due to physical (or environmental) limitations.

Code **(Note: Use intermediate codes when appropriate, e.g., 45, 68, 72.)**

100/91 Superior functioning in a wide range of activities, life's problems never seem to get out of hand, is sought out by others because of his or her many positive qualities. No symptoms.

90/81 Absent or minimal symptoms (e.g., mild anxiety before an exam), good functioning in all areas, interested and involved in a wide range of activities, socially effective, generally satisfied with life, no more than everyday problems or concerns (e.g., an occasional argument with family members).

80/71 If symptoms are present, they are transient and expectable reactions to psychosocial stressors (e.g., difficulty concentrating after family argument), no more than slight impairment in social, occupational, or school functioning (e.g., temporarily falling behind in schoolwork).

70/61 Some mild symptoms (e.g., depressed mood and mild insomnia) OR some difficulty in social, occupational, or school functioning (e.g., occasional truancy, or theft within the household), but generally functioning pretty well, has some meaningful interpersonal relationships.

60/51 Moderate symptoms (e.g., flat affect and circumstantial speech, occasional panic attacks) OR moderate difficulty in social, occupational, or school functioning (e.g., few friends, conflicts with peers or co-workers).

50/41 Serious symptoms (e.g., suicidal ideation, severe obsessional rituals, frequent shoplifting) OR any serious impairment in social, occupational, or school functioning (e.g., no friends, unable to keep a job).

40/31 Some impairment in reality testing or communication (e.g., speech is at times illogical, obscure, or irrelevant) OR major impairment in several areas, such as work or school, family relations, judgment, thinking, or mood (e.g., depressed man avoids friends, neglects family, and is unable to work; child frequently beats up younger children, is defiant at home, and is failing at school).

30/21 Behavior is considerably influenced by delusions or hallucinations OR serious impairment in communication or judgment (e.g., sometimes incoherent, acts grossly inappropriately, suicidal preoccupation) OR inability to function in almost all areas (e.g., stays in bed all day; no job, home, or friends).

20/11 Some danger of hurting self or others (e.g., suicide attempts without clear expectation of death; frequently violent; manic excitement) OR occasionally fails to maintain minimal personal hygiene (e.g., smears feces) OR gross impairment in communication (e.g., largely incoherent or mute).

10/1 Persistent danger of severely hurting self or others (e.g., recurrent violence) OR persistent inability to maintain minimal personal hygiene OR serious suicidal act with clear expectation of death.

0 Inadequate information.

The rating of overall psychological functioning on a scale of 0–100 was operationalized by Luborsky in the Health-Sickness Rating Scale (Luborsky, L. "Clinicians' Judgments of Mental Health." *Archives of General Psychiatry* 7:407–417, 1962). Spitzer and colleagues developed a revision of the Health-Sickness Rating Scale called the Global Assessment Scale (GAS) (Endicott J., Spitzer R.L., Fleiss J.L., Cohen J.: "The Global

Assessment Scale: A Procedure for Measuring Overall Severity of Psychiatric Disturbance." *Archives of General Psychiatry* 33:766–771, 1976). A modified version of the GAS was included in DSM-ILL-R as the Global Assessment of Functioning (GAF) Scale.

LEGAL ISSUES

The American Nurses Association's (ANA) *Scope and Standards of Psychiatric–Mental Health Nursing Practice* (2000) as well as the ANA *Code of Ethics for Nurses* (2001) mandate that nurses protect clients' rights. In order to do so, nurses must be aware of a wide range of client rights, the use of a psychiatric advance directive in respecting client rights, the nurse's duties to warn, to intervene, and to report abuse, and the commitment and hospitalization issues that affect client rights.

CLIENT RIGHTS

There is no one standard mental health client's bill of rights at the national level, and the variability among individual states is great. Some states guarantee several important rights; some states guarantee only a few. It is critical to safe practice to be knowledgeable about the mental health statutes and regulations in the state in which you practice. Most mental health facilities and law libraries maintain copies of mental health statutes. You may also refer to the agency in your state that oversees mental health care. In effect, mental health consumers should have the following rights.

Right to Informed Consent

A person has the right to understand and participate in the treatment process prior to consenting to treatment.

- Required by all states
- Encourages autonomy and sound decision-making
- Basic principle is client self-determination
- Competency is a key element (the person must be cognitively able to understand the problem, the negative and positive effects of the proposed treatment, and the likely outcome with and without treatment)
- Offer information the person needs in order to make an informed decision
- Assess the person's understanding of the proposed treatment

- Provide the opportunity to ask questions or gain a second opinion
- Document informed consent in writing (in a form provided by the agency or in the medical record)
- If the person lacks the ability to offer consent, determine who can advocate for the client (relative, friend, legal counsel, individual identified in a Psychiatric Advance Directive as discussed later in this section)

Right to Treatment

Depriving a person of liberty for the purpose of therapy, and then failing to provide adequate therapy violates the rights of citizens guaranteed by the U.S. Constitution. This right ensures that a person is not in a treatment setting for custodial purposes only. The necessary elements in a treatment-oriented program are:

- Physical examination and psychosocial assessment on admission, and then as indicated
- Treatment plans with clear objectives and interventions
- Client participation in treatment planning and consent for all treatment methods
- Up-to-date medical records
- Treatment in as normal an environment as possible
- Staff in adequate numbers and with sufficient training to provide quality care
- Availability of treatment that meets client needs as identified in the treatment plan
- Necessary support services such as dental, speech, physical, and rehabilitation therapy
- Ongoing treatment plan evaluations
- Programs to help clients develop skills needed for independent versus institutional living
- Adequate planning for discharge to a less restrictive setting, according to client needs

Right to Refuse Treatment

A person has a right not to be subjected to symptomatic treatments or behavioral control measures against the person's will.

- Overriding a client's right to refuse treatment is legally complicated

- If written consent is withheld by a legally incompetent person, the situation is referred to a client advocate or the client's legal counsel
- A person has the right to refuse psychotropic medications
- Most state statutes specify that electroconvulsive therapy (ECT) and psychosurgery can be administered only if informed consent is obtained from the client
- Emergency situations—usually those that involve a danger to self or others—may, in many states, override a client's right to refuse treatment

Right to Treatment in the Least Restrictive Setting

The least restrictive setting or least restrictive alternative refers to the placement of clients in the therapeutic setting that will provide care while allowing maximum freedom.

- By extension, it also means providing for the least amount of limitation or interference in an individual's thought and decision-making, physical activity, and sense of self, as necessary to provide for safety
- The ANA Standards of Psychiatric-Mental Health Nursing Practice (2000) and the American Psychiatric Nurses Association position statement on the use of seclusion and restraint (2000) expect that the nurse will choose the least restrictive limit and use it only for as long as necessary for the safety of the client and others
- Treatment settings are evaluated on such criteria as the limitations placed on physical freedom (locked versus unlocked), choice of activities, and the presence of "adult status" as shown by locked bedrooms and the unsupervised use of private bathroom facilities
- Institutional policies are evaluated as to the degree of restriction imposed by rules and regulations necessary to run the facility
- The methods sanctioned to enforce the facility's rules are evaluated for the presence of coercion or threat of punishment
- The standard for socially acceptable behavior should be no higher in the facility than it would be in the client's own environment
- Treatment is evaluated for the extent of its intrusiveness—ECT and psychosurgery are considered more intrusive than medica-

tion; long-acting medication such as fluphenazine decanoate would be considered more intrusive than oral medication

- Seclusion should be used only to prevent harm to self or others
- The use of seclusion must be documented in the person's medical record

Right to Communicate with Others

The basis for laws granting communication rights is that such communication can expose cases of wrongful hospitalization.

- Communication is unrestricted or guaranteed to named public officials or the central hospital agency for the state
- Most states extend this guarantee to include correspondence with attorneys
- Any correspondence limitation should be part of the person's clinical record
- Approximately one-half of the states require that the client has reasonable access to writing materials and postage
- Hospital authorities are generally given broad discretionary powers to curtail visitation
- Before implementing any restriction in communication or visitation, ask: Is it fair and reasonable? Could I defend it to a noninvolved professional?

Right Not to Be Subjected to Unnecessary
Mechanical Restraints

Mechanical or physical restraints restrict a person's constitutional right to liberty.

- Most states specify that restraints can be used only when the person presents a risk of harm to self or others
- Restraints are not to be used for punishment or staff convenience
- Agency policies regarding the use of restraints must be consistent with state regulations
- The use of restraints must be documented in the client's medical record

Right to Privacy

The right to privacy refers to the mental health consumer's right to keep personal information secret.

- In order for disclosure of information to occur to insurance companies, or health maintenance organizations; uninvolved staff members, mental health care students and faculty; support staff; family; lawyer; and law enforcement agencies, the client must sign a release form
- To be a valid release, the client must be told as specifically as possible what information is to be released, who needs it, why they need it, and how it will be used
- Written consent is not required for involved treatment team members; staff supervisors; involved mental health care students and faculty; and mental health care consultants
- In emergency situations (the client is in an automobile accident, has taken an overdose, is suicidal, or unable to take care of him- or herself, for example), the release of information can occur without the client's approval
- Document a breach of confidentiality, even in an emergency situation or when acting to warn/protect another or report abuse
- Instructors, students, supervisors, or team members who receive information about a client in the course of supervision or in providing treatment are also obligated to treat this material as confidential
- Reading of a medical record by someone not directly involved in the client's treatment is a breach of the client's right to privacy

Privileged communication. Protecting possibly incriminating disclosures made by clients to specified professionals is established by statute in most states.

- Has traditionally existed between husband and wife, attorney and client, clergy and church member, and physician and client (and psychologist and client in some states)
- Only a few states recognize privileged communication between client and nurse
- The privilege is the client's and can be claimed only when an established relationship is in existence
- Professionals can reveal information at the client's request.
- Each state that grants a privilege also specifies exceptions to that privilege such as some or all of the following:
  1. When acting in the client's best interests in an emergency

2. When acting to protect third parties
3. During commitment proceedings
4. When making a court-ordered evaluation or report
5. When a client has been deemed incompetent and consent is given by a guardian, or when the guardian is not available
6. When reporting child abuse, gunshot wounds, or contagious diseases, as required by state law
7. During criminal proceedings
8. In child custody disputes
9. During child abuse proceedings
10. When a client introduces a defense of mental illness into litigation proceedings

Right to Periodic Review

Periodic review provides some protection for the individual against spending more time than necessary confined to a hospital.   •
Review is required every 30 days in some states, and up to a year in others.

- In most states, short-term commitment is the rule and court review is necessary to extend commitment for another short period.

Right to Independent Psychiatric Examination

Mental health consumers have the right to an independent psychiatric assessment by a physician of their own choosing. The client must be released if the physician determines the client is not mentally ill.

Right to Participate in Legal Matters

Mental health clients have rights to participate as citizens in legal matters.

- The right to make a valid *contract* is protected unless the client has been judged legally incompetent
- A person with a psychiatric diagnosis can make a valid *will* as long as the person is aware of making a will, is familiar with the property being disposed of, and knows the names, identities, and relationships of the people named in the will
- A valid *marriage* contract hinges on the individual's possession of sufficient mental capacity to give consent (that is, that the person understands the nature of the marriage relationship

and knows the duties and obligations involved). Some states prohibit marriage while in a mental institution

- Most states have provisions for *annulment or divorce* on the grounds of prenuptial mental disability
- Most states do not prohibit the hospitalized client's right to *vote*, and some states specifically preserve this right by legislation
- States have various restrictions on *driving privileges*. Some states will not issue a driver's license to mentally disturbed people, people with epilepsy and alcohol and/or drug addiction; some states suspend driver's licenses upon admission to a mental institution; other states base suspension on legal competency

Right to Practice a Profession

Most states have some statutes prohibiting the practice of a profession by a mentally disturbed person.

- The right is impaired simply by the nature of physical confinement to a hospital
- It is usually up to professional licensing boards to suspend or revoke the license of an individual believed to be too mentally incapacitated to practice a profession safely, even though not hospitalized

Right to Habeas Corpus

The right to the speedy release of any person who has been illegally detained is protected in all states by the U.S. Constitution. Any client can petition for release on the grounds of being sane. If found sane in a hearing, the client must be discharged from the mental facility.

Rights of Children or Minors

In most states, an individual is considered a minor if younger than 18 years of age

- As a minor, a person is considered legally incompetent, and legal consent for medical treatment must come from parents or a guardia
- Exceptions to this rule include the rights to seek treatment for drug abuse, consent to contraception, and seek psychiatric treatment

- Parents can admit a child to a psychiatric facility without the child's consent, provided medical standards for admission have been met
- Some states require the consent of the child or provide for a court hearing if the child protests

DUTY TO INTERVENE, TO WARN OR PROTECT, AND TO REPORT

Duty to Intervene

In psychiatric–mental health nursing, it is often difficult to determine when and how to intervene in particular situations. The following list will help you to make this determination.

- As a nurse you form a contract for care (the client has a need for help and you agree to act in good faith for the interest of the client) when you accept the duty to care for a client
- Once a situation has come to your attention, it is important that you take all reasonable and prudent actions to be helpful to the client
- You must make a good faith effort to perform a thorough assessment of a client before intervening
- If the client is unable to cooperate in the assessment, obtain information from other sources (records from previous hospitalizations, family members, community therapists) with the client's permission
- The duty to intervene requires that information be communicated clearly to others, particularly those who participate in the decision-making process, within the established protocols of the agency of employment
- It is vital to formulate a plan before making a decision to intervene—carefully think through options and assess the clinical and legal implications of actions in a methodical fashion

Duty to Warn or Protect

An exception to confidentiality occurs with the "duty to warn" and the "duty to protect."

- The mental health care professional is responsible to balance confidentiality to the client with protection of the public from the violent client when the professional has the reasonable belief that the client is dangerous toward another

- Mental health professionals must take action to protect potential victims, especially when the individual in danger can be identified, by notifying the police and the intended victim, when possible

- Although the client has the right to confidentiality, it must be weighed against the public's need for safety from violent assault, especially when an individual in danger can be identified

Duty to Report

Another exception to confidentiality occurs with the duty to report abuse.

- Since Congress passed the National Child Abuse Prevention and Treatment Act in 1974, many states have enacted laws requiring professionals to report the abuse of minors to the police, department of social services, or child protective services.

- In many states, child abuse must be reported within 36 hours of its discovery

- Mental health professionals are not required to have evidence of abuse before reporting; the suspicion that it exists is sufficient

- Failure to report suspected abuse may have dire consequences for the minor, and the professional can be fined and/or formally reprimanded

- Protecting minors from harm is also an ethical obligation

- Most states also have an adult protective services program that responds to reports of abuse of the elderly (any adult over 65 years of age)

- In many states, elder abuse (or suspicion of it) must be reported

- Elder abuse includes theft of money or assets and neglect or abandonment, as well as physical abuse

- Safeguarding clients requires the ethical, and in some states, legal duty to report any illegal, immoral, or unethical activities of peers, including impairment through addiction to alcohol or narcotics or through an event of personal experience with emotional illness

- Be sure that you are familiar with the reporting laws in the state in which you practice

PSYCHIATRIC ADVANCE DIRECTIVE

Modeled after advance directives for end-of-life care, a psychiatric advance directive (PAD) is a mental health contingency plan which provides written direction for ethically sensitive judgment on the part of family members, significant others, professionals, and surrogates (even in states in which they are not legally recognized) for future psychiatric care.

- Respects a person's autonomy by allowing an individual to register preferences for any future psychiatric intervention
- Increases the likelihood that the person's choices will be honored
- Is legally recognized in only a few states; however, all states have a provision for a durable power of attorney for health care to which a PAD can be attached
- A written PAD allows a person to:
  1. Register refusal of psychiatric interventions such as ECT, psychotropic medications, psychosurgery, and the like
  2. Register consent and desire for specific psychiatric interventions
  3. Specify the conditions under which these interventions are acceptable
  4. Appoint a trusted surrogate decision-maker, a person(s) authorized to give consent on the individual's behalf
  5. Register willingness or unwillingness to participate in psychiatric research studies
  6. Register who should be notified about admission to a psychiatric facility, who should be prohibited from visiting, and who should have temporary custody of children
  7. Improve communication between the person and the mental health care provider
  8. Possibly shorten a hospital stay and/or reduce the use of court proceedings

COMMITMENT AND HOSPITALIZATION

There is great variability in commitment and hospitalization procedures from state to state. Be sure to know the law in the state in which you practice.

- *Voluntary admission* comes about by written application for admission by prospective clients, or someone acting in their behalf. The client has a right to demand and obtain release, after giving notice (usually in writing) during a grace period of from 24 hours to 15 days, depending on the state

- *Informal voluntary admission* is an option in several states, in which the client verbally requests admission and is free to leave the facility at any time

- *Involuntary commitment* refers to the state's ability to hospitalize an individual involuntarily. All state involuntary commitment procedures include one or more of the following criteria—dangerous to self or others (the only justification in an increasing number of states), unable to provide for basic needs, mentally ill. Can be in one of four categories—emergency, temporary or observational, extended or indeterminate, and outpatient

- *Involuntary outpatient commitment* has been used to ensure that individuals follow through with outpatient treatment once released from a mental health facility or a prison, and to prevent further deterioration of the person's mental health that would require inpatient hospitalization

PROTECTING YOURSELF LEGALLY

- Be aware of provisions in your state nurse practice act
- Follow standards of care
- Know the relevant law
- Review agency procedures and policies with both the standards of care and relevant law in mind, clarify any conflict with legal counsel if necessary, and then follow procedures
- Practice protective documentation (see pp. 205–206)
- Question the physician about any ambiguous orders before carrying them out
- Be sure to carry your own malpractice insurance

STANDARD PRECAUTIONS

The Centers for Disease Control and Prevention have developed a set of precautions designed to prevent the transmission of human immunodeficiency virus (HIV), hepatitis B virus (HBV), and other bloodborne pathogens when providing health care. All blood is assumed to be potentially infective. Standard precautions apply to:

- Blood
- Body fluids containing visible blood
- Semen and vaginal secretions
- Cerebrospinal fluid (CSF)
- Synovial fluid
- Pleural fluid
- Peritoneal fluid
- Pericardial fluid
- Amniotic fluid

Standard precautions do not apply to feces, nasal secretions, sputum, sweat, tears, urine, vomitus, and human breast milk unless they contain visible blood. The risk of transmission of HIV and HBV from these fluids is extremely low or nonexistent.

Standard precautions are not intended to replace hand washing as routine infection control. The precautions supplement hand washing through the utilization of protective barriers to reduce the risk of exposure of the nurse's skin or mucous membranes. Protective barriers include gloves, gowns, masks, and protective eyewear. The type of protective barrier is determined by the procedure being performed and the anticipated type of exposure. Gloves should be worn for touching blood and body fluids requiring standard precautions, mucous membranes, or nonintact skin of all clients. Gloves should also be worn for handling items or surfaces contaminated with blood or body fluids to which standard precautions apply. Gloves should be changed after contact with each client and hands should be washed immediately after gloves are removed. Gloves cannot prevent penetrating injuries caused by the mishandling of needles, scalpels, and other sharp instruments. Sharp items are to be placed in puncture-resistant containers marked with a biohazard symbol for disposal.

Masks and protective eyewear or face shields should be worn by health care workers to prevent exposure of the mucous membranes of the mouth, nose, and eyes during procedures that are likely to create droplets of blood or body fluids. Gowns should be worn during procedures that are likely to generate splashes of blood or body fluids (CDC, 1988; National Institutes of Health, 2001).

THE NURSING PROCESS

ASSESSMENT

The nursing process begins with assessment for the purpose of collecting and analyzing objective and subjective data about the clients.

NEUROPSYCHIATRIC ASSESSMENT

Assessing clients on their neuropsychiatric status involves focusing on a number of different facets of their lives. How clients function, their capabilities of interacting with others, their effectiveness in various settings and what those settings consist of, are all included in the neuropsychiatric assessment.

Psychosocial Assessment

Psychosocial assessment is a dynamic process that begins during the initial contact with the client and continues throughout the nurse–client experience. Psychosocial assessments may be made of an individual, or may be completed on a family or a group. In any case, they begin with the identifying characteristics, such as name, sex, age, marital status, and ethnic and cultural origins. Problem identification and definition are also necessary phases in the assessment process.

During the individual assessment, you consider the following factors in significant detail:

1. Physical and intellectual functioning
2. Socioeconomic factors
3. Personal values and goals
4. Adaptive functioning and response to present involvement
5. Developmental factors

Psychologic Testing

Clinical psychologists administer and interpret a wide variety of psychologic tests. There are two types of psychologic tests: those concerned with intelligence and those concerned with personality. Both intelligence and personality tests are typically included in a comprehensive psychologic evaluation.

Intelligence tests may be useful particularly in evaluating the presence and degree of mental retardation and to assess cognitive functioning. Personality tests are objective and projective. Objective personality tests provide data on various aspects of the client's personality, which is scored or analyzed using empirically derived criteria. Projective personality tests involve presenting the client with a somewhat ambiguous stimulus, often a visual one, to which the client responds with an idiosyncratic perception: for example, the client states what the stimulus looks like or makes up a story about it. It is thought that in this process the client projects something of herself or himself into the response.

Rorschach Test.   An example of a projective personality test is the Rorschach Test. Hermann Rorschach, a Swiss psychiatrist, developed the Rorschach Test in 1921 that consists of ten standardized inkblots in black and white or color on separate cards, displayed one by one. Clients are asked to respond in terms of their associations, thoughts, and impressions. Because each card contains only inkblots, clients' responses are thought to be projections of important aspects of their inner psychodynamic functioning. The examiner scores the responses according to:

- *Location.* Where on the blot area was the response seen?
- *Determinant.* What characteristic of the blot prompted the response?
- *Content.* What did the client see?
- *Form-level.* How closely did the response correspond to the contour of the blot area used?
- *Originality.* How common a response is it?

Interpretation is based on a complicated system of scoring responses and analyzing content. In recent years, there have been efforts to develop empirically based systems of content analysis to enable greater standardization of Rorschach scoring and interpretation.

Thematic Apperception Test (TAT).   The Thematic Apperception Test (TAT) also consists of a series of cards shown one by one, but the TAT cards are pictures of people in various situations. Clients are asked to describe what seems to be happening in the picture, what the people are feeling and thinking, and how the situation that is seen will be resolved. Because the pictures are ambiguous, the responses are thought to reveal aspects of the clients' own emotional lives. The psychologist who interprets and scores the TAT looks for themes, threads, and patterns in the responses. Some adaptations of the TAT for use with children are available.

The Wechsler Adult Intelligence Scale-III (WAIS-III).   An example of a cognitive function test is the Wechsler Adult Intelligence Scale-III (WAIS-III), which consists of 14 subtests which permit the derivation of verbal IQ score, performance IQ score, full scale IQ score, and four specialized indices of specific areas of cognitive functioning. Most frequently only 11 subtests which are necessary and sufficient for the derivation of IQ scores are administered. In addition to providing information on the verbal and nonverbal (performance) abilities of the client, comparisons between individual subtest scores can be evaluated to yield data on relative specific cognitive strengths and weaknesses of the client.

Raven's Progressive Matrices Test. The Raven's Progressive Matrices Test is designed to provide data on intellectual ability in a relatively culturally unbiased manner. Many other intelligence tests depend on knowledge and skills that are somewhat culturally bound. The Raven's Progressive Matrices Test asks the client to solve two-dimensional visual–spatial items of increasing difficulty, items that are relatively culturally unbiased. Scores on this test can be translated into empirically derived categories of intellectual ability.

Benton Visual Retention Test. The Benton Visual Retention Test is an example of a neuropsychological assessment instrument that can yield valuable data on aspects of a person's cognitive functioning. It is sometimes used as a quick screening device to see if the test-taker may be manifesting signs of cognitive dysfunction. It is more often used to provide details on the nature of cognitive dysfunction being manifested by someone who has already been determined to have a cognitive problem or difficulty. The test-taker is asked to reproduce various geometric designs after examining the designs for a few seconds. The type and frequency of different kinds of errors, as well as the number of designs reproduced correctly, are compared with empirically based frequency tables to determine the extent to which cognitive dysfunction may be possible, probable, or strongly indicated. The test performance is strongly influenced by any difficulties in the test-taker's visual processing, organization, memory, and visual–motor skills.

The Mental Status Examination (MSE). The mental status examination (MSE) is usually a standardized procedure. The primary purpose of the MSE is to help the examiner gather more objective data to be used in determining etiology, diagnosis, prognosis, and treatment, and to deal immediately with any risk of violence or harm. The sections of the mental status examination that deal with sensorium and intellect are particularly important in establishing the existence of delirium, dementia, amnestic, and other cognitive disorders. The purpose of this examination differs from that of a psychiatric history in that it identifies the person's present mental status.

You will generally seek the following categories of information, not necessarily in the sequence presented here.

1. **General behavior, appearance, and attitude.** A complete and accurate description of the client's physical characteristics, apparent age, manner of dress, use of cosmetics, personal hygiene, and responses to you. Postures, gait, gestures, facial expression, and mannerisms are included in the description. Also note the client's general activity level. Other descriptors could be "frank," "friendly," "irritable," "dramatic," "evasive," "indifferent," and so forth. Details should be sufficient to identify and characterize the client.

2. **Characteristics of talk.** The form, rather than the content, of the client's speech is described in terms of loudness, flow, speed, quantity, level of coherence, and logic. A sample of the client's conversation with you may be included in quotation marks. The goal is to describe the quantity and quality of speech to discern difficulties in thought processes. The following patterns, if present, should be particularly noted.
   a. *Mutism.* No verbal response despite indications that the client is aware of your questions.
   b. *Circumstantiality.* Cumbersome, convoluted, and unnecessary detail in response to your questions.
   c. *Perseveration.* A pattern of repeating the same words or movements despite apparent efforts to make a new response.
   d. *Flight of ideas.* Rapid, overly productive responses to questions that seem related only by chance associations between one sentence fragment and another. Patterns you may observe with flight of ideas might be rhyming, clang associations, punning, and evidence of distractibility.
   e. *Blocking.* A pattern of sudden silence in the stream of conversation for no obvious reason.

3. **Emotional state.** The person's pervasive or dominant mood or affective reaction. Both subjective and objective data are included. Subjective data are obtained through the use of non-leading questions, for instance, "How are you feeling?" If the client replies with general terms, such as "nervous," ask the

client to describe how the nervousness shows itself and its effect, since such words may mean different things to different individuals. Observe objective signs, such as facial expression, motor behavior, the presence of tears, flushing, sweating, tachycardia, tremors, respiratory irregularities, states of excitement, fear, and depression. The attitude of the client toward you sometimes offers valuable clues. Attitudes of hostility, suspiciousness, or flirtatiousness, a desire for bodily contact, or outspoken criticisms should be noted.

The psychiatric client is apt to have a persistent emotional trend reflective of a particular emotional disorder, such as depression. If this is true, probe further to discover the intensity and persistence of this reaction, in keeping with DSM-IV-TR criteria.

It is desirable to record verbatim the replies to questions concerning the client's mood. The relationship between mood and the content of thought is particularly significant. There may be a wide divergence between what clients say or do and their emotional state as expressed by attitudes or facial expressions.

Note whether intense emotional responses accompany discussion of specific topics. Shallowness or flat affect is indicated by an insufficiently intense emotional display in association with ideas or situations that ordinarily would call for a stronger response. Dissociation or disharmony is often indicated by an inappropriate emotional response, such as smiling or silly behavior, when the attitude should be one of concern, anxiety, or sadness. It is difficult to evaluate emotional reactions in clients who use simulation or play-acting. Clients who are trying to cover up a deep depression may feign cheerfulness and good spirits. The client's emotional reactions may be constant or may fluctuate during the examination. Try to specify the ease or readiness with which such changes occur in response to pleasant or unpleasant stimuli. The following terms can be used to describe intensity of response:

- Composed, complacent, frank, friendly, playful, teasing, silly, cheerful, boastful, elated, grandiose, ecstatic
- Tense, worried, anxious, pessimistic, sad, perplexed, bewildered, gloomy, depressed, frightened
- Aloof, superior, disdainful, distant, defensive, suspicious
- Irritable, resentful, hostile, sarcastic, angry, furious
- Indifferent, resigned, apathetic, dull, affectless

Pay attention to the influence of content on affect, and note disharmony between affect and content or thought and whether the emotional state is constant or changes.

4. **Content of thought:** *special preoccupations and experiences.* Delusions, illusions, or hallucinations, depersonalizations, obsessions or compulsions, phobias, fantasies, and daydreams. You can elicit these data by asking such questions as, "Do you have any difficulties?" or "Have you been troubled or ill in any way?"

Delusions are false beliefs. If the client has delusions of being the object of environmental attention, some of the following questions might reveal them: "Do people like you?" "Have you ever been watched or spied upon or singled out for special attention?" "Do others have it in for you?" *Delusions of alien control* (passivity) are feelings of being controlled or guided by external forces. If you suspect these delusions, ask the client such questions as, "Do you ever feel your thoughts or actions are under any outside influences or control?" "Are you able to influence others, to read their minds, or to put thoughts in their minds?"

A client with *nihilistic delusions* more or less completely denies reality and existence. The client states that nothing exists, or that everything is lost. Statements such as "I have no head, no stomach," "I cannot die," or "I will live to eternity" suggest nihilistic delusions.

Delusions of self-deprecation are often seen in connection with severe depressions. The client describes feeling unworthy, sinful, ugly, or foul smelling.

Delusions of grandeur are associated with elated states such as great wealth, strength, power, sexual potency, or identification with a famous person or a god.

Somatic delusions are focused on having cancer, obstructed bowels, leprosy, or some horrible disease. These are to be distinguished from a preoccupation with normal, visceral, or peripheral sensations.

Hallucinations are false sensory impressions with no external basis in fact. Try to elicit the clearness of the projection to the outside world—for example, the source of the voices (from outside or inside the head), the clarity and distinctness of the perception, and the intensity. Be subtle in approaching the client for evidence of hallucinatory phenomena, unless the client is obviously hallucinating. In the case of obvious hallucinations, it's appropriate to ask about them directly.

Obsessions are insistent thoughts recognized as arising from the self. The client usually regards them as absurd and relatively meaningless, yet they persist despite endeavors to get rid of them. *Compulsions* are repetitive acts performed through some inner need or drive and supposedly against the client's wishes, yet not performing them results in tension and anxiety.

Fantasies and daydreams are preoccupations that are often difficult to elicit from the client. The difficulty may be that the client misunderstands what you want, but often people are ashamed to talk about their fantasies and daydreams because of their content.

5. **Orientation.** Orientation in terms of time, place, person, and self or purpose to determine the presence of confusion or clouding of consciousness. You may introduce such questions by asking, "Have you kept track of the time?" If so, "What is today's date?" Clients who say they don't know should be asked to estimate approximately or to guess at an answer. Many clinicians begin the mental status exam with these questions because disorientation should cause the examiner to question the validity and reliability of data obtained subsequently.

6. **Memory.** The person's attention span and ability to retain or recall past experiences in both the recent and the remote past. If memory loss exists, determine whether it is constant or variable and whether the loss is limited to a certain time period. Be alert to *confabulations*—invented memories to take the place of those the client cannot recall. It is useful to introduce questions relating to memory by some general statement such as "Has your memory been good?" or "Have you had difficulty remembering telephone numbers or appointments?"

   a. *Recall of remote past experiences.* Ask for a review of the important events in the client's life. Then compare the response with information obtained from other sources during the history taking.

   b. *Recall of recent past experiences.* These are events leading to the present seeking of treatment.

   c. *Retention and recall of immediate impressions.* You might ask the client to repeat a name, an address, or a set of objects (for example, rose, teacup, and battleship) immediately and again after 3–5 minutes. Another test is to have the client repeat three-digit numbers at a rate of one per second, or to repeat a complicated sentence.

     d. *General grasp and recall.* You might ask the client to read a story and then repeat the gist with as many details as possible.

7. **General intellectual level.** A nonstandardized evaluation of intelligence. The examiner looks for the person's ability to use factual knowledge in a comprehensive way.

     a. *General grasp of information.* You may ask the client to name the five largest cities of the United States, the last four presidents, or the governor of the state.

     b. *Ability to calculate.* Tests of simple multiplication and addition are useful for this purpose. Another test consists of subtracting from one hundred by sevens until the person can go no further (serial sevens test).

     c. *Reasoning and judgment.* A common test of reasoning is to ask clients what they might do with a gift of $10,000. You must be particularly careful to correct for your own biases and values in assessing each client's answer.

8. **Abstract thinking.** The distinctions between such abstractions as poverty and misery or idleness and laziness. It is common to ask the client to interpret simple fables or proverbs, like "Don't cry over spilled milk."

9. **Insight evaluation.** Whether clients recognize the significance of the present situation, whether they feel the need for treatment, and how they explain the symptoms. Often it is helpful to ask clients for suggestions for their own treatment.

10. **Summary.** The important psychopathologic findings and a tentative diagnosis. Any pertinent facts from the medical history and/or physical examination should be added to the summary.

    Mini-Mental State Exam (MMSE).   It is possible to fairly accurately assess and evaluate a client's functioning in a streamlined manner. The Mini-Mental State Exam (MMSE) provides a framework for such an assessment. These 11 questions cover the scope of the way a client thinks and reacts. There are scores assigned to each question and the total score indicates the likelihood and level of cognitive decline.

    For the test to be efficient and valid you must ask the questions in the order in which they are listed. The main focus of the examination is cognitive functioning, although the client's mood can be ascertained in the process. The maximum score is 30 points and the score is represented as a fraction with the actual points scored as the numerator and 30 points as the denominator (i.e., 28/30, 20/30, etc.). It is important to note that there are limitations to using the MMSE with people who have certain disabilities with sight or motor movement allowing writing. If a client is not able to perform one of the activities, it may be necessary to conduct a full mental status exam or to document the results of the relevant aspects of the MMSE without a score.

Physiologic Assessment

Nurses must carefully consider the possibility that a client's symptoms may have a physiologic, biologic, or in particular, a neurologic basis. In some reported instances, clients with brain tumors or bromide intoxication or nutritional deficiencies have been hospitalized on psychiatric units and treated exclusively for their seemingly psychiatric symptoms. Such a critical oversight obviously delays and seriously hampers appropriate treatment of the correct biologic or neurologic problem. The value of careful assessment regarding general health issues and screening for biologic disorders cannot be overemphasized. In many community settings, psychiatric–mental health nurses are the only mental health care providers prepared to undertake a biologic and neurologic assessment and interpret the results.

The objectives of a biologic and neurologic assessment are:

1. Detection of underlying and perhaps unsuspected organic disease that may be responsible for psychiatric symptoms
2. Understanding of disease as a factor in the overall psychiatric disability
3. Appreciation of somatic symptoms that reflect primarily psychologic rather than physiologic problems

Since the client's history is essential to the process of physiologic assessment, inquire into three primary areas of biologic history:

1. Facts about known physical diseases and dysfunction
2. Information about specific physical complaints
3. General health history

Previous Illnesses. Information about previous illnesses may provide essential clues. Clients with comorbidities of substance abuse and mental disorder are particularly challenging. For example, suppose the presenting symptoms include paranoid delusions and the client has a history of similar episodes. During each previous episode, the client responded to various forms of treatment and demonstrated no residual symptoms. This history suggests a strong possibility of amphetamine- or other drug-related psychosis, and a drug screen laboratory test may be indicated. An occupational history may provide information about exposure to inorganic mercury, leading to symptoms of psychosis; or exposure to lead, resulting in mental disorder.

Specific Physical Complaints.   The second area of emphasis in biologic history taking is eliciting information from the client about specific physical complaints. Again, it is crucial for the nurse to consider symptoms in terms of both psychiatric conditions and physical diseases. Symptoms that are atypical of psychiatric disorders are particularly revealing clues. For example, suppose a client with hallucinations and delusions also complains of a severe headache at the onset of the symptoms. The symptoms together suggest possible brain disease and call for careful and repeated neurologic assessment and use of brain imaging techniques.

History-taking should also include information about the medications the client is currently taking. Digitalis intoxication may result in impairment. Reserpine may produce symptoms generally considered psychiatric in nature.

General Health History.   The third area is that of the general health history. As mentioned above, psychiatric nurses need to be able to assess for a variety of general health problems and therefore need to have medical-surgical nursing skills. Keep in mind that some medical problems are masked by psychiatric symptoms, and psychiatric symptomatology can be the result of a medical disorder. Observation also yields important data bearing on the possible presence of organic disorders.

- An unsteady gait may suggest diffuse brain disease or alcohol or drug intoxication.
- Asymmetry—dragging a leg or not swinging one arm—might be a sign of a focal brain lesion.
- Although inattention to proper hygiene and dress, particularly mismatched socks or shoes, is common in people with emotional disorders, it is also a hallmark of dementias.
- Frequent, quick, purposeless movements are characteristic of anxiety, but they are equally characteristic of chorea and hyperthyroidism.
- Tremors accompanied by anxiety may point to Parkinson's disease.

- Recent weight loss, although often encountered in depression and schizophrenia, may be due to gastrointestinal disease, carcinoma, Addison's disease, and many other physical disorders.

You should observe skin color, pupillary changes, alertness and responsiveness, and quality of speech and word production, keeping in mind the possibility of delirium, dementia, substance intoxication, or other medical conditions.

Family Assessment

Assessing and intervening with families of your clients is an essential role. The family who has cared for the client with a mental disorder has an in-depth understanding of the client's illness, history, and ability to function in the community. Include the family's insights in the assessment phase, and, if appropriate, use them in the planning of care, particularly care after discharge.

Family assessment involves gathering data in several different areas and can be done both formally and informally. Do not overlook natural opportunities to assess families and their needs. During visits, join the family for a few minutes to learn about their understanding of the treatment program, their concerns, and their questions. More formal assessments using interview guides or strategies such as a family genealogy or time line (discussed later in this chapter) are also available. Whichever methods you use, remember that a trusting relationship with key members of the client's family is essential for establishing a flow of information and planning care. Remember, however, to secure clients' permission before information is released to their families, and encourage clients to involve their families in their treatment (Marshall & Solomon, 2000).

Demographic Information.   Data pertaining to gender, age, occupation, religion, and ethnicity should be obtained. In addition to gathering discrete bits of information (the father is a 39-year-old Latino, physician's assistant, and a member of St. Ann's Roman Catholic parish), it is important to gather more detailed information that will give insight into family functioning.

- How actively does the family pursue religious/spiritual activities?
- What is the link of religion/spirituality to the family's value system, norms, and practices?

- What is the family's racial, cultural, and ethnic identification in relation to sense of identity and belonging?
- Who in the family is employed?
- What are their attitudes about employment?

Past Medical and Mental Health History.   Here, substantive information should also be gathered. You will want to know about past medical and mental health treatment; past and present illnesses; and pertinent health facts in the family of origin, the extended family, and in the family history.

- Gather information about the developmental stage of the family—what were (are) the problems in transition from one developmental level to another?
- How has the family solved problems at earlier stages?
- What shifts in role responsibility have occurred over time?

Family Interactional Data.   This is probably the most complex data to obtain. For example, you will want to gather information about family rules.

- What family rules foster stability in the family? What rules foster maladaptation?
- How are rules modified?
- What happens when all members do not agree about the family rules?

You will also need to determine the roles of family members.

- What are the formal roles for each member? What are the informal roles (scapegoat, controller, decision-maker, and so on)?
- Do the roles seem to have a good fit in the family?
- How do family members communicate? What are the channels of communication—who speaks to whom?
- Are the messages clear? What is the extent of unclear or ambiguous messages, mixed messages, or missed messages?
- Do members "hear" one another?

Assess levels of cohesion by noting who accompanies the client during admission. Visits from family are a rich source of information.

- Does the whole family visit, or just one member?

- Does the client come in alone?
- Who visits, how often, and for how long?
- How do family visitors behave with the client? Do the members spend time interacting and sharing activities, do they sit quietly together, or do they maintain physical and emotional distance from one another?

Document these patterns of family interactions, and monitor the effect of family visits on the client.

Family Burden.   Most families of mentally disordered individuals report that caring for the ill member is a very important, largely underappreciated, and frequently expensive, all-consuming, and lifelong task (Karp, 2000). *Family burden* is a term that refers to the difficulties and responsibilities of family members who assume a caretaking function for relatives with psychiatric disability. Family burdens reported most often are financial strain, violence in the household, reductions in the physical and mental health of family caregivers, disruption in family routines, worry about the future, the impact of stigma, the mental health system itself as a stressor, and feeling overwhelmed or unable to cope. Gathering information about the family burden will help you to determine such things as:

- What kind of support would be most helpful to this family? A family support group? Referral to the National Alliance for the Mentally Ill (NAMI)?
- Respite care to give the family a break from their caregiving role?
- Family therapy?

Family System Data.   How does the family interact with the outside world? How permeable or rigid are its boundaries? Find out the extent to which the family fits into the larger culture of which it is a part. To what degree could the family be considered deviant from the larger culture?

Within the family, what are the family alliances—who supports whom? Which members are in conflict with one another, or with the family as a whole? Are there extended family supports? What other social supports are available to the family?

Needs, Goals, Values, and Aspirations.   Determine whether essential physical needs are met. At what level does the family meet the social and emotional needs of its members? What are the individual needs of family members, and how do they fit with the family needs? Is the family willing or able to meet the individual needs of its members?

Determine the extent to which individual family members' goals and values are articulated and understood by the other members. Are the goals and values shared by all? Do some members compromise? Do other members simply give up and give in? Does the family as a whole allow individual members to pursue individual goals and values?

Cultural Assessment

Knowledge empowers us to understand cultural differences. Sensitivity enables us to respect and honor differences. Sensitivity and knowledge must be combined with skills for accurate assessment and effective nursing interventions.

Communication is crucial to all nursing care, but it is especially important when caring for mental health clients from diverse backgrounds. To establish contact, present yourself in a confident way without seeming to be superior. Shake hands, if appropriate. Allow clients to choose their comfortable personal space. Respect their version of acceptable eye contact. Ask how they prefer to be addressed. Most people are pleased when others show sincere interest in them.

You may have to learn to use certain indirect styles of communication and wait to see if and how the client responds. Observe how the client communicates to others to learn what style is most appropriate. Storytelling is a valuable approach to sharing views. Inviting clients to tell you stories about themselves and their problems is an excellent way to find out what is important to them and how they view their situations. "Can you tell me a story about when you were growing up?" "Would you tell me a story about coming to the hospital/clinic?" Communication is most productive when you acknowledge that clients know more about their personal situation than you do. Having clients tell the story of their life and of their illness often provides information that will help you understand their experiences and views. Although this approach requires good listening skills and adequate amounts of time, it forms the core of effective professional practice.

Cultural assessment questions include:

- Where were you born?
- Where were your parents born?
- Describe your contact and closeness with extended family members.

- Do you live in a neighborhood where many families are of the same ethnic background?
- Describe the type of ethnic activities that are important to you.
- Tell me what you heard about people with mental illness when you were growing up.
- Did your family or friends consider people with mental illness to be evil, possessed, bizarre, weak, sick, dangerous, or incompetent?
- What do you believe causes mental illness?
- What led you to seek treatment at this time?
- In what ways have you experienced discrimination because of your mental illness?

Lack of understanding often leads to moral judgments about people who are labeled mentally ill. Cultural attitudes determine how people with mental illness are treated. Condemning stereotypes often keep individuals from seeking treatment and this contributes to their feeling ashamed of needing treatment. The effects of stigma and discrimination are often more damaging than the day-to-day struggles of living with an impairment.

Spiritual Assessment

Spirituality is that part of us that deals with relationships and values, and addresses questions of purpose and meaning in life. Spirituality unites people and is inclusive in nature, not exclusive. Although spirituality is not a religion, being involved in a particular religion is a way some people enhance their spirituality. Yet people can be very spiritual and not religious. Spirituality involves individuals, family, friends, and community. Assessment questions include:

- What do you think is the purpose of your life?
- Describe the role of illness in your life.
- What is your view of death?
- In what ways does fear, anger, guilt, or worry interfere with your sense of peace?
- Describe your sense of hope at this time.
- In what way are all humans the same and connected to one another?
- In what ways do you feel connected to family members and/or friends?

- Under what circumstances do you feel lonely?
- In what way, if any, do you feel connected to an external power often identified as God, a Supreme Being, or the Great Mystery?
- Describe how you think life is fair or unfair to most people, including yourself.
- Do you belong to a religious group?
- Do you participate in any spiritual activities such as meditating or praying, religious activities, mystical experiences, self-help groups, caring for others, or enjoying nature?
- Do you have a spiritual advisor you would like to contact at this time?

People's spiritual health is expressed through humor, compassion, faith, forgiveness, courage, and creativity. Spirituality enables us to develop healthy relationships based on acceptance, respect, and compassion.

DIAGNOSIS

Analysis of the significance of the assessment data results in the formulation of nursing diagnoses. Standardized labels are applied to clients' problems and responses to mental disorders. These standardized labels come from the list of approved nursing diagnoses accepted by the North American Nursing Diagnosis Association (NANDA). The following is the current list of approved diagnoses:

2003–2004 NANDA-APPROVED NURSING DIAGNOSES

Activity Intolerance

Activity Intolerance, Risk for

Adaptive Capacity: Intracranial, Decreased

Adjustment, Impaired

Airway Clearance, Ineffective

Anxiety

Anxiety, Death

Aspiration, Risk for

Attachment, Parent/Infant/Child, Risk for Impaired

Body Image, Disturbed

Body Temperature: Imbalanced, Risk for

Bowel Incontinence

Breastfeeding, Effective

Breastfeeding, Ineffective

Breastfeeding, Interrupted

Breathing Pattern, Ineffective

Cardiac Output, Decreased

Caregiver Role Strain

Caregiver Role Strain, Risk for

Communication, Readiness for Enhanced

Communication: Verbal, Impaired

Confusion, Acute

Confusion, Chronic

Constipation

Constipation, Perceived

Constipation, Risk for

Coping: Community, Ineffective

Coping: Community, Readiness for Enhanced

Coping, Defensive

Coping: Family, Compromised

Coping: Family, Disabled

Coping: Family, Readiness for Enhanced

Coping (Individual), Readiness for Enhanced

Coping, Ineffective

Decisional Conflict (Specify)

Denial, Ineffective

Dentition, Impaired

Development: Delayed, Risk for

Diarrhea

Disuse Syndrome, Risk for

Diversional Activity, Deficient

Dysreflexia, Autonomic

Dysreflexia, Autonomic, Risk for

Energy Field, Disturbed

Environmental Interpretation Syndrome, Impaired

Failure to Thrive, Adult

Falls, Risk for

Family Processes, Dysfunctional: Alcoholism

Family Processes, Interrupted

Family Processes, Readiness for Enhanced

Fatigue

Fear

Fluid Balance, Readiness for Enhanced

Fluid Volume, Deficient

Fluid Volume, Deficient, Risk for

Fluid Volume, Excess

Fluid Volume, Imbalanced, Risk for

Gas Exchange, Impaired

Grieving, Anticipatory

Grieving, Dysfunctional

Growth, Disproportionate, Risk for

Growth and Development, Delayed

Health Maintenance, Ineffective

Health Seeking Behaviors (Specify)

Home Maintenance, Impaired

Hopelessness

Hyperthermia

Hypothermia

Identity: Personal, Disturbed

Infant Behavior, Disorganized

Infant Behavior: Disorganized, Risk for

Infant Behavior: Organized, Readiness for Enhanced

Infant Feeding Pattern, Ineffective

Infection, Risk for

Injury, Risk for

Knowledge, Deficient (Specify)

Knowledge (specify), Readiness for Enhanced

Latex Allergy Response

Latex Allergy Response, Risk for

Loneliness, Risk for

Memory, Impaired

Mobility: Bed, Impaired

Mobility: Physical, Impaired

Mobility: Wheelchair, Impaired

Nausea

Neurovascular Dysfunction: Peripheral, Risk for

Noncompliance (Specify)

Nutrition, Imbalanced: Less than Body Requirements

Nutrition, Imbalanced: More than Body Requirements

Nutrition, Imbalanced: More than Body Requirements, Risk for

Nutrition, Readiness for Enhanced

Oral Mucous Membrane, Impaired

Pain, Acute

Pain, Chronic

Parenting, Impaired

Parenting, Readiness for Enhanced

Parenting, Risk for Impaired

Perioperative Positioning Injury, Risk for

Poisoning, Risk for

Post-Trauma Syndrome

Post-Trauma Syndrome, Risk for

Powerlessness

Powerlessness, Risk for

Protection, Ineffective

Rape-Trauma Syndrome

Rape-Trauma Syndrome: Compound Reaction

Rape-Trauma Syndrome: Silent Reaction

Relocation Stress Syndrome

Relocation Stress Syndrome, Risk for

Role Conflict, Parental

Role Performance, Ineffective

Self-Care Deficit: Bathing/Hygiene

Self-Care Deficit: Dressing/Grooming

Self-Care Deficit: Feeding

Self-Care Deficit: Toileting

Self-Concept, Readiness for Enhanced

Self-Esteem, Chronic Low

Self-Esteem, Situational Low

Self-Esteem, Risk for Situational Low

Self-Mutilation

Self-Mutilation, Risk for

Sensory Perception, Disturbed (Specify: Visual, Auditory, Kinesthetic, Gustatory, Tactile, Olfactory)

Sexual Dysfunction

Sexuality Patterns, Ineffective

Skin Integrity, Impaired

Skin Integrity, Risk for Impaired

Sleep Deprivation

Sleep Pattern Disturbed

Sleep, Readiness for Enhanced

Social Interaction, Impaired

Social Isolation

Sorrow, Chronic

Spiritual Distress

Spiritual Distress, Risk for

Spiritual Well-Being, Readiness for Enhanced

Spontaneous Ventilation, Impaired

Sudden Infant Death Syndrome, Risk for

Suffocation, Risk for

Suicide, Risk for

Surgical Recovery, Delayed

Swallowing, Impaired

Therapeutic Regimen Management: Community, Ineffective

Therapeutic Regimen Management, Effective

Therapeutic Regimen Management: Family, Ineffective

Therapeutic Regimen Management, Ineffective

Therapeutic Regimen Management, Readiness for Enhanced

Thermoregulation, Ineffective

Thought Processes, Disturbed

Tissue Integrity, Impaired

Tissue Perfusion, Ineffective (Specify type: renal, cerebral, cardiopulmonary, gastrointestinal, peripheral)

Tissue Perfusion, Ineffective (Peripheral)

Transfer Ability, Impaired

Trauma, Risk for

Unilateral Neglect

Urinary Elimination, Impaired

Urinary Elimination, Readiness for Enhanced

Urinary Incontinence, Functional

Urinary Incontinence, Reflex

Urinary Incontinence, Stress

Urinary Incontinence, Total

Urinary Incontinence, Urge

Urinary Incontinence, Risk for Urge

Urinary Retention

Ventilatory Weaning Response, Dysfunctional

Violence: Other-Directed, risk for

Violence: Self-Directed, risk for

Walking, Impaired

Wandering

Source: NANDA Nursing Diagnoses: Definitions and Classification, 2003-2004. Philadelphia: North American Nursing Diagnosis Association. Used with permission.

PLANNING

Planning consists of identifying outcome criteria and goals to assist the client toward a higher level of functioning and improved mental health.

OUTCOME IDENTIFICATION: NOC*

The widespread use of NANDA's nursing diagnoses has increased awareness of the need for standardized classifications of nursing outcomes. Outcomes are positive or negative changes in

---

*Reprinted from *Nursing Outcomes Classification*, M. Johnson and M. Maas, 2nd edition, (2000), with permission from Elsevier Science.

health status that can be credited to nursing care. They allow us to evaluate the appropriateness of our decision-making process in selecting nursing interventions. Outcomes are important for the quality of nursing care and clinical evaluation research. Nursing Outcomes Classification (NOC) is a list of standardized measures that reflect the current status of clients. Outcomes are descriptive, on a continuum from the least desirable to the most desirable states of behaviors. Goals, on the other hand, are prescriptive— the state or behavior you want the client to achieve. Outcomes tell you where the client is at any given moment, and goals tell you where you want the client to end up (Johnson, Maas, & Moorhead, 2000).

NOC is a three-level taxonomy. The highest level contains seven *domains* (or supercategories):

1. Functional Health
2. Physiologic Health
3. Psychosocial Health
4. Health Knowledge and Behavior
5. Perceived Health
6. Family Health
7. Community Health

Each domain includes *classes* (or subcategories), which are groups of general outcomes. The third level in the taxonomy has more specific outcomes. Third-level outcomes have specific indicators that nurses use to determine the client's status. The following is an example of the NOC taxonomy:

DOMAIN: Psychosocial Health

CLASS: Psychological Well-Being

Outcomes: *Hope*
  Definition
  Presence of internal state of optimism that is personally satisfying and life-supporting
  Scale
  5-point scale from none to extensive
  Indicators
  (Sample from a list of 13 indicators)
  • Expression of a positive future orientation
  • Expression of will to live

- Expression of reasons to live
- Expression of meaning in life
- Expression of inner peace

The following are examples of outcomes that are most appropriate to psychiatric–mental health nursing.

DOMAIN: Physiologic Health

CLASS: Neurocognitive

Outcomes

Cognitive ability:
Ability to execute complex mental processes

Cognitive orientation:
Ability to identify person, place, and time

Communication ability:
Ability to receive, interpret, and express spoken, written, and nonverbal messages

Concentration:
Ability to focus on a specific stimulus

Decision-making:
Ability to choose between two or more alternatives

Information processing:
Ability to acquire, organize, and use information

DOMAIN: Psychosocial Health

CLASS: Psychological Well-Being

Outcomes

Body image:
Positive perception of own appearance and body functions

Depression level:
Severity of melancholic mood and loss of interest in life events

Hope:
Presence of internal state of optimism that is personally satisfying and life-supporting

Identity:
Ability to distinguish between self and non-self and to characterize one's essence

Loneliness:
The extent of emotional, social, or existential isolation response

Mood equilibrium:
Appropriate adjustment of prevailing emotional tone in response to circumstances

Self-esteem:
Personal judgment of self-worth

Sexual identity—Acceptance:
Acknowledge and acceptance of own sexual identity

Will to live:
Desire, determination, and effort to survive

CLASS: *Psychosocial Adaptation*

Outcomes

Acceptance—health status:
Reconciliation to health circumstances

Coping:
Actions to manage stressors that tax an individual's resources

Grief resolution:
Adjustment to actual or impending loss

Psychosocial adjustment—life change:
Psychosocial adaptation of an individual to a life change

CLASS: *Self-Control*

Outcomes

Abusive behavior self-control:
Self-restraint of own behaviors to avoid abuse and neglect of dependents or significant others

Aggression control:
Self-restraint of assaultive, combative, or destructive behavior toward others

Anxiety control:
Personal actions to eliminate or reduce feelings of apprehension and tension from an unidentifiable source

Depression control:
Personal actions to minimize melancholy and maintain interest in life events

Distorted thought control:
Self-restraint of disruption in perception, thought processes, and thought content

Fear control:
Personal actions to eliminate or reduce disabling feelings of alarm aroused by an identifiable source

Impulse control:
Self-restraint of compulsive or impulsive behaviors

Self-mutilation restraint:
Ability to refrain from intentional self-inflicted injury

Substance addiction consequences:
Compromise in health status and social functioning due to
substance addiction

Suicide self-restraint:
Ability to refrain from gestures and attempts at killing self

CLASS: *Social Interaction*

Outcomes

Role performance:
Congruence of an individual's role behavior with role expectations

Social interaction skills:
An individual's use of effective interaction behaviors

Social involvement:
Frequency of an individual's social interactions with persons,
groups, or organizations

Social support:
Perceived availability and actual provision of reliable assistance from other persons

DOMAIN: *Health Knowledge and Behavior*

CLASS: *Health Knowledge*

Outcomes

Knowledge—diet:
Extent of understanding conveyed about diet

Knowledge—medications:
Extent of understanding conveyed about medication

Knowledge—substance use control:
Extent of understanding conveyed about managing substance
use safely

CLASS: *Risk Control and Safety*

Outcomes

Risk control—alcohol use:
Actions to eliminate or reduce alcohol use that poses a threat
to health

Risk control—drug use:
Actions taken to eliminate or reduce drug use that poses a threat to health

DOMAIN: Perceived Health

CLASS: *Health & Life Quality*

Outcomes

Quality of life:
An individual's expressed satisfaction with current life circumstances

Spiritual well-being:
Personal expressions of connectedness with self, others, higher power, all life, nature, and the universe that transcend and empower the self

Suffering level:
Severity of anguish associated with a distressing symptom, injury, or loss with potential long-term effects

Well-being:
An individual's expressed satisfaction with health status

DOMAIN Family Health

CLASS: *Family Caregiver Status*

Outcomes

Caregiver–patient relationship:
Positive interactions and connections between the caregiver and care recipient

CLASS: *Family Member Health Status*

Outcomes

Abuse cessation:
Evidence that the victim is no longer abused

Abuse protection:
Protection of self or dependent others from abuse

Abuse recovery—emotional:
Healing of psychologic injuries due to abuse

Abuse recovery—financial:
Regaining monetary and legal control or benefits following financial exploitation

Abuse recovery—physical:
Healing of physical injuries due to abuse

Abuse recovery—sexual:
Healing following sexual abuse or exploitation

Caregiver emotional health:
Feelings, attitudes, and emotions of a family care provider while caring for a family member or significant other over an extended period of time

Neglect recovery:
Healing following the cessation of substandard care

Once you have established outcomes, you and the client mutually identify goals for change. Mutual goal-setting is the process of collaborating with clients to identify and prioritize care goals and develop a plan for achieving those goals. Underlying this process is respect for clients' cultural values. You begin by assessing the clients' degree of insight into their problems. If clients are too acutely ill to be actively involved in the initial goal formulation, or if they are in denial of mental health problems, they must at least be informed of the goals and given an opportunity to express their opinions (McCloskey & Bulechek, 2000).

Clients are encouraged to identify strengths and abilities that they bring to this problem-solving process. You help them identify realistic, attainable goals and break down complex goals into small, manageable steps. After goals become manageable, work with clients on prioritizations so they try to modify only one behavior at a time. Finally, help clients develop a plan to meet their goals which includes identifying available resources, setting realistic time limits, and clarifying the roles of the nurse and client. Regular review dates are established with clients and families to review progress toward outcomes and goals (McCloskey & Bulechek, 2000).

IMPLEMENTATION

Caring is a way of relating to people that enables them to grow toward their full potential. Your nursing interventions should be implemented in a manner that recognizes the worth and dignity of people and considers the physical, emotional, social, cultural, and spiritual needs of your clients and their families.

NURSING INTERVENTIONS CLASSIFICATION: NIC*

Once the nursing diagnoses, outcome criteria, and goals have been identified, the plan of care is developed to assist the client toward a higher level of functioning and improved mental health. The Nursing Interventions Classification (NIC) is a standardized classification of nursing interventions for use with individuals, families, and communities.

NIC is a three-level taxonomy. The highest level contains six *domains* (or supercategories):

1. Physiological: Basic
2. Physiological: Complex
3. Behavioral
4. Safety
5. Family
6. Health System

Each domain includes classes (or subcategories) that are groups of related interventions. The third level in the taxonomy is the interventions. Supplementing the interventions is a list of nursing activities for each intervention. This is not a list of specific procedures as not all activities apply to every client. In addition, nurses may modify or add to the list of activities. The following is an example of the NIC taxonomy:

DOMAIN: Behavioral

CLASS: *Coping Assistance*

Intervention *Hope instillation*

Definition Facilitation of the development of a positive outlook in a given situation.

Activities (Sample from a list of 18 activities)
- Assist patient/family to identify areas of hope in life
- Expand the patient's repertoire of coping mechanisms
- Help the patient expand spiritual self
- Encourage therapeutic relationships with significant others
- Provide patient/family opportunity to be involved with support groups

---

*Reprinted from *Nursing Interventions Classifications,* J.C. McCloskey and G.M. Bulecheck, 3rd editon, (2000), with permission from Elsevier Science.

The following are examples of interventions that are most appropriate to psychiatric–mental health nursing (McCloskey & Bulechek, 2000):

DOMAIN: Physiological: Basic

CLASS: Activity and Exercise Management

Interventions *Exercise promotion:* Facilitation of regular physical exercise to maintain or advance to a higher level of fitness and health

CLASS: Elimination Management

Interventions *Constipation management:* Prevention and alleviation of constipation

CLASS: Immobility Management

Interventions *Physical restraint:* Application, monitoring, and removal of mechanical restraining devices or manual restraints which are used to limit physical mobility of patient

CLASS: Nutritional Support

Interventions *Eating disorders management:* Prevention and treatment of severe diet restriction and overexercising, or binging and purging of food and fluids

Nutritional management: Assisting with or providing a balanced dietary intake of food and fluids

CLASS: Physical Comfort Promotion

Interventions *Progressive muscle relaxation:* Facilitating the tensing and releasing of successive muscle groups while attending to the resulting differences in sensation

Simple massage: Stimulation of the skin and underlying tissues with varying degrees of hand pressure to decrease pain, produce relaxation, and improve circulation.

CLASS: Self-Care Facilitation

Interventions *Self-care assistance:* Assisting another to perform activities of daily living

Sleep enhancement: Facilitation of regular sleep–wake cycles

DOMAIN: Behavioral

CLASS: Behavioral Therapy

Interventions *Activity therapy:* Prescription of and assistance with specific physical, cognitive, social, and spiritual activities to increase the range, frequency, or duration of an individual's (or group's) activity

Animal-assisted therapy: Purposeful use of animals to provide affection, attention, diversion, and relaxation

Art therapy: Facilitation of communication through drawings or other art forms

Assertiveness training: Assistance with the effective expression of feelings, needs, and ideas while respecting the rights of others

Behavior management—overactivity: Provision of a therapeutic milieu which safely accommodates the patient's overactivity while promoting optimal function

Behavior management—self-harm: Assisting the patient to decrease or eliminate self-mutilating or self-abusive behaviors

Behavior management—sexual: Delineation and prevention of socially unacceptable sexual behaviors

Behavior modification: Promotion of a behavior change

Behavior modification—social skills: Assisting the patient to develop or improve interpersonal social skills

Limit setting: Establishing the parameters of desirable and acceptable patient behavior

Milieu therapy: Use of people, resources, and events in the patient's immediate environment to promote optimal psychosocial functioning

Music therapy: Using music to help achieve a specific change in behavior or feeling

Mutual goal setting: Collaborating with a patient to identify and prioritize care goals, then developing a plan for achieving those goals through the construction and use of goal attainment scaling

Patient contracting: Negotiating an agreement with a patient that reinforces a specific behavior change

Play therapy: Purposeful use of toys or other equipment to assist a patient in communicating his/her perception of the world and to help in mastering the environment

Self-responsibility facilitation: Encouraging a patient to assume more responsibility for own behavior

Substance use prevention: Prevention of an alcoholic or drug use life style

Substance use treatment: Supportive care of patient/family members with physical and psychosocial problems associated with the use of alcohol or drugs

Substance use treatment—alcohol withdrawal: Care of the patient experiencing sudden cessation of alcohol consumption

Substance use treatment—drug withdrawal: Care of a patient experiencing drug detoxification

Substance use treatment—overdose: Monitoring, treatment, and emotional support of a patient who has ingested prescription or over-the-counter drugs beyond the therapeutic range

CLASS: *Cognitive Therapy*

Interventions *Anger control assistance:* Facilitation of the expression of anger in an adaptive nonviolent manner

Cognitive restructuring: Challenging a patient to alter distorted thought patterns and view self and the world more realistically

Reality orientation: Promotion of patient's awareness of personal identity, time, and environment

Reminiscence therapy: Using the recall of past events, feelings, and thoughts to facilitate adaptation to present circumstances

CLASS: *Communication Enhancement*

Interventions *Active listening:* Attending closely to and attaching significance to a patient's verbal and nonverbal messages

Socialization enhancement: Facilitation of another person's ability to interact with others

CLASS: *Coping Assistance*

Interventions *Anticipatory guidance:* Preparation of patient for an anticipated developmental or situational crisis

Coping enhancement: Assisting a patient to adapt to perceived stressors, changes, or threats which interfere with meeting life demands and roles

Counseling: Use of an interactive helping process focusing on the needs, problems, or feelings of the patient and significant others to enhance or support coping, problem solving, and interpersonal relationships

Crisis intervention: Use of short-term counseling to help the patient cope with a crisis and resume a state of functioning comparable to or better than the pre-crisis state

Grief work facilitation: Assistance with the resolution of a significant loss

Guilt work facilitation: Helping another to cope with painful feelings of responsibility, actual or perceived

Mood management: Providing for safety and stabilization of a patient who is experiencing dysfunctional mood

Recreation therapy: Purposeful use of recreation to promote relaxation and enhancement of social skills

Self-esteem enhancement: Assisting a patient to increase his or her personal judgment of self-worth

Spiritual support: Assisting the patient to feel balance and connection with a greater power

Therapy group: Application of psychotherapeutic techniques to a group, including the utilization of interactions between members of the group

CLASS: *Patient Education*

Interventions *Teaching—disease process:* Assisting the patient to understand information related to a specific disease process

CLASS: *Psychological Comfort Promotion*

Interventions *Anxiety reduction:* Minimizing apprehension, dread, foreboding, or uneasiness related to an unidentified source of anticipated danger

Calming technique: Reducing anxiety in patient experiencing acute distress

Distraction: Purposeful focusing of attention away from undesirable sensations

Simple guided imagery: Purposeful use of imagination to achieve relaxation and direct attention away from undesirable sensations

Simple relaxation therapy: Use of techniques to encourage and elicit relaxation for the purpose of decreasing undesirable signs and symptoms such as pain, muscle tension, or anxiety

DOMAIN: Safety

CLASS: *Crisis Management*

Interventions *Rape-trauma treatment:* Provision of emotional and physical support immediately following an alleged rape

Suicide prevention: Reducing risk of self-inflicted harm for a patient in crisis or severe depression

CLASS: *Risk Management*

Interventions *Abuse protection:* Identification of high-risk, dependent relationships and actions to prevent further infliction of physical or emotional harm

Abuse protection—child: Identification of high-risk, dependent child relationships and actions to prevent possible or further infliction of physical, sexual, or emotional harm or neglect of basic necessities of life

Abuse protection—elder: Identification of high-risk, dependent elder relationships and actions to prevent possible or further infliction of physical, sexual, or emotional harm, neglect of basic necessities of life, or exploitation

Area restriction: Limitation of patient mobility to a specified area for purposes of safety or behavior management

Delirium management: Provision of a safe and therapeutic environment for the patient who is experiencing an acute confusional state

Delusion management: Promoting the comfort, safety, and reality orientation of a patient experiencing false, fixed beliefs that have little or no basis in reality

Dementia management: Provision of a modified environment for the patient who is experiencing a chronic confusional state

Elopement precautions: Minimizing the risk of a patient leaving a treatment setting without authorization when departure presents a threat to the safety of patient or others

Hallucination management: Promoting the safety, comfort, and reality orientation of a patient experiencing hallucinations

Seclusion: Solitary containment in a fully protective environment with close surveillance by nursing staff for purposes of safety or behavior management

DOMAIN: Family

CLASS: *Life Span Care*

Interventions *Caregiver support:* Provision of the necessary information, advocacy, and support to facilitate primary patient care by someone other than a health care professional

Family involvement: Facilitating family participation in the emotional and physical care of the patient

Family mobilization: Utilization of family strengths to influence patient's health in a positive direction

Family therapy: Assisting family members to move their family toward a more productive way of living

PSYCHOEDUCATION

Education of consumers and families is basic to nursing care. Knowledge empowers people to make informed decisions regarding their health status, plan for maintaining wellness, and illness care choices.

Education in the mental health care setting involves more than giving information to passive people. Education is an active process that is done with people, not to people. The steps of the nursing process are used in the educational process: assessing the learning needs, diagnosing the knowledge deficit with contributing factors, planning content, implementing the most effective methods of education, evaluating the effectiveness of the teaching, and documenting the entire process.

Assertiveness

There are a number of ways someone can react to a situation: passive, aggressive, passive-aggressive, and assertive. See the diagram below for one view of these reactions and interactions.

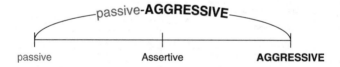

A passive response shows fear and does not allow an individual to take his or her own needs into account. An aggressive response shows anger and only takes the individual's needs into account while discounting or abusing others' needs. A passive-aggressive response shows passive and submissive behavior but beneath this façade is a great deal of hostility and resentment. The assertive response respects one's own needs and the needs of others. It does not depend on fear or anger, but promotes communication and problem-solving. The example below demonstrates these responses.

There are three basic components of an assertive response:

1. Start the response with "I," as opposed to "You," "They," or any other word.
2. Describe the situation as you see it. Include your feelings if appropriate to the situation (work situations may need a description of the situation without your personal feelings being detailed).
3. Suggest a solution to the problem.

    Note that the passive, passive-aggressive, and aggressive responses can result in problematic communication and/or relationship difficulties.

Leenie is extremely busy and stressed at work, especially lately. She belongs to a professional organization that meets monthly, rotating among the members' homes. Leenie gets a call at work from Charlene, the organization's president and a close personal friend of Leenie's, regarding the next meeting.

Charlene: "Hi, Leenie. We all decided that your cooking was the greatest and so our next meeting is going to be at your house in two weeks. All 17 of us are expecting one of your famous gourmet meals, too. Got to go. Bye."

Passive response	Leenie does not want to clean her house and cook this big meal, but she decides it wouldn't be that bad if she did a little bit every day between now and the meeting.
Aggressive response	Leenie calls Charlene back and says loudly and angrily, "I wouldn't feed you and your rabble any of my cooking if you were the last people on earth. Take your meeting and all those ridiculous goofs and go bother someone else."
Passive-aggressive response	Leenie cooks barely enough for 10 people, saying Charlene specifically told her that only 10 people would be attending.
Assertive response	Leenie calls Charlene back. Leenie asks if Charlene has a minute to talk about the meeting: "I feel overwhelmed lately and I don't think a gourmet dinner would work out. How about if everyone comes to my house for a meeting and brings along a favorite dish to share?"

Conflict Management

Disagreement and conflict in family, friendship, and work relationships are normal. The problem is not that people disagree, but that they do not know how to resolve their differences. Teaching clients general principles for resolving conflict is a helpful nursing intervention. The following are eight steps to resolve interpersonal disagreements.

1. *Stay calm.* When people are calm, they think much more clearly. Calmness is difficult to maintain when people call each other names, become sarcastic, or drag up past injustices. Do not try to solve problems when people are very angry.

2. *Express commitment to the relationship.* Arguments often leave people feeling like enemies rather than family members, friends, or co-workers. It is important to defuse that by saying, "I care about you (or the job). Let's work together to work this problem out."

3. *Identify areas of agreement or success.* Teach people to look for similarities in their viewpoint or find positive characteristics in the other person. People who are in conflict often get stuck on arguing about one small point and overlook that they agree on many other points.

4. *Identify the specific problem.* It is difficult to resolve problems when arguments keep escalating with the addition of more and more problems.

5. *Express the desired outcome.* People should clearly state what they want to happen so that everybody is clear about each other's goals.

6. *Listen carefully to the other person's concerns.* Each person needs to hear what the other is saying. If necessary, have them repeat the essence of what they heard to show that they understand. Problems cannot be solved if individuals are planning what they are going to say next, rather than listening carefully to what is being said to them.

7. *Seek solutions that benefit the relationship.* Teach individuals to brainstorm possible solutions and how to look for ways to compromise and meet everyone's needs.

8. *Assess the outcome.* Teach people to analyze the solution before it is implemented. Has everyone felt respected and heard? Is everyone at least partially satisfied with the

solution? If so, the conflict has probably been resolved successfully.

Family and Parenting Skills

Individuals with mental illness often have family members who share in the many losses that accompany the illness. Families are the major source of support and rehabilitation for their loved ones. Of clients discharged from acute care, 65 percent return to their families. At any given time, 40 to 50 percent of the 48 million Americans who are psychiatrically disabled live with their families on a regular basis. Even when consumers do not live at home, their families are often the only source of support. Care for the mentally ill has become as much family based as community based in the United States. This situation can result in overwhelming emotional and economic stress on the family system.

Family members are often the first to notice that their family member is exhibiting unusual behavior. As it becomes more evident that there is a significant problem, families begin to search for reasons and solutions. Families begin to develop their own image of the disease process and expectations of mental health professionals. Many families also hope for what was in the past and for what might be in the future. The expectation of a meaningful and productive individual and family life is shattered. All family members must be supported as they grieve the loss of their hopes and dreams.

Families must be supported in their day-to-day efforts to cope with all the changes in the family. When people become psychiatrically disabled, they often find they cannot carry out their family roles and responsibilities. Thus, other family members must assume those role functions and come to terms with an altered family lifestyle. They must develop cognitive, emotional, and behavioral coping strategies to be able to live with their loved one who is experiencing a mental disorder. Some of these strategies include:

- Expressing affection
- Suggesting alternative choices
- Reducing conflict
- Focusing on the positive parts of the relationship with the disabled family member.
- Seeking social support from friends and family
- Finding spiritual support

- Seeking professional support and community resources
- Becoming active in the National Alliance for the Mentally Ill (NAMI), an organization of consumers, families, and professionals.

Pregnancy and Child Care. Pregnancy, childbirth, and parenting are major issues for all women. For the psychiatrically disabled woman, who already has problems in adjustment and coping, pregnancy and parenting can cause sufficient strain to exacerbate symptoms of the mental illness. Women with a history of mental illness must be monitored closely throughout their pregnancy. Many pregnancies are unplanned and it is not uncommon for women and their families to be unaware of a pregnancy until the pregnancy is far advanced, which places both the woman and fetus at risk. Other problems may include a diminished ability to comply with prenatal care, an inability to plan realistically for the baby, an increased risk of substance abuse during the pregnancy, and poor nutrition. The woman may also feel overwhelmed and ambivalent about motherhood and may fear losing custody of the baby.

Psychiatric disability among mothers of newborns and young children has far-reaching implications for the mother and the family. If the mother is acutely ill at childbirth, she is usually separated from her newborn, which may be deeply distressing for her and impede the bonding process. This separation may be temporary, but in some cases the loss of custody becomes permanent. Psychiatric hospitalization for acute illness leads to disruption of the family system as children suffer repeated separations and a chaotic and unpredictable environment.

Nursing interventions for young families include helping the family develop a social support system and use community resources. Teaching includes providing information about normal growth and development, stress-management techniques, time-management skills, and problem-solving skills. Collaborating with the extended family may minimize the impact of psychiatric disability on the primary family.

Youth. An estimated 8 million children (12 to 13 percent of all children under age 18) have a serious emotional disturbance with substantial functional impairment, nearly half of which leads to serious disability. Children with mental disorders are at increased risk for dropping out of school and of being marginalized members of society in adulthood. Mental disorders are seldom identified in young children.

When a child or adolescent experiences a mental disorder, the entire family system is strained. When primary responsibility for caregiving falls to one person, the parental system is stressed, which often leads to increased conflict and a greater likelihood of parental separation. The siblings are often excluded, leading to confusion or misunderstanding of the problem. Siblings' feelings many range from shame to protectiveness. At times, they may feel superior for not having "problems," while at other times they may feel neglected if the child with the disorder receives more parental attention.

The parent–child relationship is often severely strained due to stressors related to the child's mental disorder. Some parents respond in ways that foster independence, which contributes to separation/individuation problems or boundary issues. Some parents may be rejecting and critical of the child with the disorder. Other parents alternate between overprotection/overcontrol and rejection. Other families learn to adapt in ways that foster the growth and development of all the children.

Couples. Most people who are psychiatrically disabled at a fairly young age remain single. Their social functioning is so limited that they are unable to sustain a relationship. In contrast, people with mood disorders, anxiety disorders, or substance use disorders may be able to be part of a couple. Many of them, however, report serious couple difficulties and hope to resolve these relationship problems in therapy. In addition, couples who are experiencing relationship distress are at higher risk for depression, anxiety, and substance use.

Adult Children. Since at least half of the psychiatrically disabled population lives with their families on a regular basis, professionals are beginning to look at and respond to the burden of family caregivers. Some of the problems that families of these adult children face are the need for daily caretaking, lack of freedom, emotional drain, stress of the unexpected, and financial strain. Parents often struggle to find a good balance between supporting their adult child with an illness as a dependent and fostering her or his own independence to the greatest extent possible. This balance involves both the person with the disability and the caregiving parent.

Client symptoms of illness such as inappropriate behavior, labile emotions, hallucinations, delusions, and outbursts of rage are often difficult for families to manage. Other symptoms that strain the family are dependency, poor social skills and outlets, and difficulty finding employment. Parents are often concerned about the welfare of their child after their death. Family caregivers need support and practical knowledge to enhance their ability to cope and their ability to support their loved one.

Vulnerability to Relapse

Understandably, families are very concerned with their loved one's vulnerability to relapse. Although families are not to be blamed for mental disorders, their interactions may influence the course of the disorder. Relapse is less common in families who see the client as ill (rather than lazy or manipulative) and provide support to one another. Relapse is more common in families who are highly critical, highly anxious, and preoccupied with their problems. Researchers have studied two family patterns: family expressed emotion (EE) and family affective style (AS). Families rated as high EE tend to be hostile, critical, and emotionally overinvolved with the client. Families rated as high AS are intrusive and make guilt-inducing remarks during emotionally charged family discussions. Both high EE and SA families are predictors of relapse for people who are psychiatrically disabled. Families are more likely to be excessively critical or overinvolved when they lack information about the disorder and when they believe the symptoms are under the client's control.

Medication noncompliance and substance abuse are other changeable factors related to relapse. Medication noncompliance is linked to lack of insight into the disorder, medication side effects, cost of medication, missed outpatient appointments, and negative client/family attitudes toward medication. Mental health status is further compromised by the use of alcohol or drugs. Clients who abuse substances also tend to be noncompliant with medication.

Problem-Solving

The most important process for clients and families to learn is how to solve problems. As they become increasingly skilled at problem solving, they will expand their coping skills and enhance the quality of their lives. In teaching the problem-solving process, focus on one problem at a time, and measure progress by observing small changes.

Because all problems are connected, changes in one problem will cause changes in others. Remind people that in the past they have done their best to deal with problems, and that new solutions may now be found. Your role is to listen, observe, encourage, and evaluate. More effective coping behavior will be the ultimate result of the problem-solving process. But before the process can begin, you must help them identify their problem. Identification includes the person's definition of the problem, the significance of the problem, and the influence of the past and future. Throughout the problem-solving process, it is extremely helpful to have clients keep a written list of all the ideas generated. The list can be modified as time goes on.

After problem identification has been completed, the steps of the problem-solving process consist of the following:

1. Identifying the solutions that have been attempted
2. Listing alternative solutions
3. Predicting the probable consequences of each alternative
4. Choosing the best alternative to implement
5. Implementing the chosen alternative in a real-life or practice situation
6. Evaluating outcomes

The first step is identifying what solutions have been tried thus far. The specifics of the attempts, how the attempts were implemented, and what occurred as a result must all be clarified. Because the problem continues to exist, these solutions were not effective, so they should be either modified or discarded.

The second step is having the client list alternative ways of solving the problem. Frequently, the client will have only one or two ideas. You can propose brainstorming sessions to increase creativity in problem solving. All possible solutions, even those that are unrealistic or absurd, are written down. Thinking of absurd solutions often opens the mind to other creative, realistic solutions to the problem. Finally, after the client has listed all his or her ideas for solving the problem, you can add your own suggestions.

The third step is predicting the probable consequences of each alternative, which helps clients anticipate outcomes of behavior. After thorough discussion, you and your client go on to the fourth step: choosing the best alternative to implement. Do not make this decision for clients; doing so would undermine the process by placing them in a childlike, dependent position. Using action-oriented terms, develop the selected solution further, as concretely and specifically as possible. At the same time, formulate measurable outcomes to use in evaluating the process.

The fifth step is implementing the proposed solution in either a practice or a real-life situation. Clients must be allowed to make mistakes during this step. If you rescue them, you are sending the message that they are incapable of taking charge of their lives.

Evaluation is the sixth step in the problem-solving process. Review the outcomes, and determine the degree of success or failure in achieving them. Successfully achieving an outcome means that the solution was effective and that it can continue to be implemented. Failing to achieve an outcome means you and your client need to analyze how and why the solution was ineffective. Then return to step 4, and either select a new solution or modify the old one.

As clients experience the steps of the problem-solving process, they increase their skills, which then can be applied to other problematic areas of life. With an improved ability to make and assume responsibility for decisions, they develop an internal locus of control, leading to competence and self-esteem.

Psychosocial Rehabilitation

The field of psychosocial rehabilitation grew out of a need to create opportunities for people suffering from psychiatric disabilities. Psychosocial rehabilitation is the development of skills and supports necessary for successful living, learning, and working in the community. This approach creates collaborative partnerships with all interested people—consumers, families, friends, and mental health care providers. Recovery, a facet of rehabilitation, refers to incorporating the disability as part of reality, modifying dreams and aspirations, exploring new ideas, and eventually adapting to the disease. Each person's road to recovery is unique. It is assumed that the consumer will be "in charge" with regard to setting goals for where and how to live, work, learn, socialize, and recreate. Rehabilitation is a process, not a quick fix. This approach is quite different from the traditional approach to long-term consumers, where the assumption was that people with psychiatric disabilities needed to have decisions made for them.

People with mental illness differ little from the general population. They want work that is meaningful and self-enhancing and the opportunity to socialize with others. Psychosocial rehabilitation is anchored in the values of hope and optimism that people can grow, learn, and make changes in their lives. One essential element is power. People who have mental disorders need power and control in their relationships with professionals, in their own lives, and in the way resources are allocated. This allows them to take personal responsibility for where they are in their lives and where they are going (Test & Stein, 2000).

As a nurse, you not only provide care, but work with clients to make decisions about treatment and about daily life. Recovery is about providing temporary support during hard times while working with clients to take responsibility for their own wellness.

Recovery is a personal choice. When you find resistance and apathy to recovery, you may feel frustrated as a nurse. It is important to recognize that severity of symptoms, motivation, and personality type can affect a person's ability to work toward recovery. Some people work at it intensely while others approach recovery more slowly. It is not up to you to determine when a person is ready to make progress—it is up to the person (Mead & Copeland, 2000).

Social Skills Training

Individuals who are psychiatrically disabled often benefit from social skills training. Community treatment focuses primarily on the teaching of basic coping skills necessary to live as autonomously as possible in the community. Inadequate social and vocational skills may force clients to remain in institutional settings. Social skills training to overcome disabilities is repetitive and lengthy, and is measured in months or years. Clients must also have opportunities and encouragement to practice social skills in real life and reinforcement for the use of these skills in community life.

Social skills training can be done in individual or group sessions. Clients have individualized behavioral goals to guide them as they empower themselves to adapt to community living. Steps in teaching social skills are:

1. Provide a rationale for learning the skill.
2. Break the skill into component steps.
3. Model the skill through role-playing.
4. Review with clients what they observed in the role play.
5. Role play with clients to practice the skill.
6. Provide positive feedback about components that were performed well.
7. Provide corrective feedback on how the skill could be done better.
8. Have clients role play the skill with other clients.
9. Have clients practice the skill at home/work.

Activities of Daily Living Skills. Activities of Daily Living (ADLs) skills include such skills as grooming and personal hygiene, room upkeep, laundry upkeep, cooking, shopping, eating at restaurants, budgeting, use of public transportation, and time management. Those clients who are severely disabled benefit from being taught in their own setting. For instance, laundry upkeep is most effectively taught in the client's neighborhood laundromat; cooking, on his/her own stove; and room cleaning in his/her own home. The inability to perform several of these basic ADLs for a length of time can create enormous frustration and stress, which may contribute to relapse.

Vocational Skills. Psychiatrically disabled clients may lack not only specific work skills, but also job-seeking abilities and good work habits. Being persistently unemployed contributes to feelings of inadequacy and low self-esteem. Clients may need support in locating positions, filling out applications, role-playing interviews, and learning job expectations and behaviors. Some community mental health centers provide job coaches if necessary; these coaches work alongside clients on the job until they can gradually be self-sufficient.

Leisure Time Skills. Some clients lack either the interest or the necessary skills to fill their free time in a satisfying manner. When clients spend the majority of their free time in solitary television viewing, they are susceptible to increasing withdrawal, with accompanying loneliness and depression often leading to gradual decompensation. Clients are encouraged to find leisure and social activities that are enjoyable and involve interaction with others. Discover what are meaningful activities for each individual as well as their preferences for activities. Help them choose activities consistent with their physical, psychological, and social capabilities. Focus on skills they have rather than on deficits. Discuss with clients the scheduling of specific periods for leisure activity into their daily routine. As with ADLs, leisure time activities should be carried out in the client's own neighborhood. Teach clients about available community resources for leisure activities (YMCA, YWCA, community center, local bowling alley, swimming pool, gym), support groups, and religious expression.

Interpersonal Skills. Without basic interpersonal skills, it is difficult to implement many of the activities just mentioned or to maintain a state of well-being. Clients need to learn how to interact appropriately with family members, friends, or strangers and at work and school. They must be able to identify and express their own feelings and respect and listen to those of others. Some will need assistance with conversational skills such as initiating conversations, asking questions, making appropriate self-disclosures, and ending conversations gracefully. Assertiveness training is appropriate for clients who are either passive or aggressive in their style of relating to others. Clients may need to learn conflict resolution skills, which involves learning compromise and negotiation skills so that conflicts with others can be worked out in a satisfactory manner. As they become increasingly skilled at problem solving, they will expand their social skills and enhance the quality of their lives.

THERAPIES

The establishment of a therapeutic alliance is fundamental to the therapeutic change process in therapy. A therapeutic alliance is a conscious relationship between a facilitative person and a client. In this process, the helping person forms a mature alliance with the growth-facilitating aspects of the client. Each implicitly agrees to work together to help the client address personal problems and concerns. A therapeutic alliance is particularly helpful when the client experiences increased anxiety during the therapy process and resistance to change.

Therapy is built upon a mutually defined, collaborative, and goal-oriented professional relationship. Most therapies have three distinct phases or stages through which they progress:

1. The orientation phase, characterized by the establishment of contact with the client
2. The working phase, characterized by the maintenance and analysis of contact
3. The termination phase, characterized by the termination of contact with the client

The length of therapy depends on several factors—primarily the needs of the client, the principles that undergird the therapy, and realistic factors such as length of hospitalization and financing. Individual, group, and family therapies may need to be adjusted, depending upon the time available; for example, a client in an inpatient setting may be there for only a few days. Stages or phases may be briefer and have less depth and intensity than longer term outpatient work.

Individual Therapy

Individual therapy, often called one-to-one relationship therapy, involves one client and one therapist. What nurses call the therapeutic nurse–client relationship is based on the principles of individual therapy and the creation of a therapeutic alliance.

Orientation Phase.   The major goal of the orientation phase of individual therapy is to establish contact and begin to form a working relationship with the client. You clarify the purpose of individual therapy, your role, and the responsibilities of the client, offering to work with the client toward the alleviation of the client's suffering. During this phase, the therapeutic contract (the client's definition of personal goals for treatment and the therapist's professional responsibilities) is negotiated.

The usual interventions in this phase include:

- Providing information regarding the purpose, role, and responsibilities in individual therapy to alleviate initial client anxiety
- Immediately and explicitly addressing any misconceptions, fantasies, and fears regarding individual therapy and the therapist
- Using facilitative personal characteristics, especially empathic understanding
- Avoiding premature reassurance (allowing trust to evolve)
- Whenever possible, encouraging the formation of goals that are specific, addressing intrapersonal and interpersonal behavioral patterns, and designating the degree of change necessary for client self-satisfaction
- Establishing the contract—place, duration, and time of therapy; client and therapist responsibilities; fees and payment intervals, if any; referral sources

Working Phase.   The working phase centers around behavioral analysis—the mutual determination of the dynamics of response patterns identified by the client, especially those considered to be dysfunctional—and achieving constructive change in behavior. Troublesome thoughts, feelings, and behaviors are addressed, and coping skills to deal with the anxiety associated with constructive changes in behavior are facilitated.

The usual interventions of this phase include:

- Exploring response patterns in depth, linking elements of one response pattern to other patterns for a gradual unfolding of central life patterns

- Increasing awareness of defenses to ward off anxiety and help the client challenge personal resistance to change
- Encouraging the client to evaluate each response pattern to determine which are self-defeating
- Facilitating the strengthening of existing growth-promoting coping skills and encouraging the development of new coping skills and their application to actual life experiences
- Creating an atmosphere offering permission for active experimentation to test and assess the effectiveness of new behaviors
- Helping the client learn and apply problem-solving strategies and active decision-making as a means to personal accountability

Termination Phase.   The goal of the termination phase is to terminate contact in a mutually planned, satisfying manner. Termination usually follows the client's relief from the symptoms that interfered with the client's comfort, the acquisition of adaptive coping strategies, and the achievement of treatment goals. The usual interventions of this phase include:

- Encouraging the client's realistic appraisal of personal therapeutic goals (motivation, effort, progress, outcome) as these evolved in treatment
- Reviewing the client's assets and therapeutic gains as well as areas for further therapeutic work
- Encouraging the transference of dependence on empathic, emotional support to other support systems (spouse, relative, friend, support group)
- Participating in an explicit therapeutic goodbye with the client
- Being alert to the surfacing of any behavior that arises on termination—repression, regression, acting-out, anger, withdrawal, and acceptance—in order to help the client work through feelings associated with these behaviors
- Allowing time and space for termination; the longer the duration of the individual therapy, the more time is needed for the termination phase

Group Therapy

Nurses have long been involved in working with clients in small groups brought together for psychoeducation or support purposes. All nurses, regardless of level of education, can lead therapeutic groups as long as they understand and apply group and therapeutic principles in their work. The role of the nurse as group therapist is reserved for advanced practice clinical specialists prepared at the master's level and above.

According to Yalom (1995), the core of group therapy is a focus on the here and now. The here-and-now work of the group therapist occurs on two levels:

1. Focusing attention on each member's feelings toward other group members, the therapist(s), and the group
2. Illuminating the process (the relationship implications of interpersonal transactions)

Thus, group members need to become aware of the here-and-now events—what happened, and then reflect back on them—why it happened.

Orientation Phase. The usual interventions of this phase include:

- Being active and providing structure and direction (suggest members introduce themselves, include all members, encourage sharing but limit monopolizing)
- Moving to reduce anxiety; avoiding making demands until group anxiety has abated
- Clarifying the contract; giving information to dispel confusion or misunderstandings
- Beginning exploration by focusing on related themes
- Beginning to focus on here-and-now experiences in sessions
- Encouraging members to become involved with others, thus facilitating the curative factor of universality

Working Phase. The usual interventions of this phase include:

- Encouraging cohesion by providing the opportunity for the expression of warm feelings
- Encouraging exploration and moving to problem-solving
- Observing and commenting on the here and now, and encouraging members to participate similarly
- Illuminating the process by making process comments (the relationship implications of interpersonal transactions)
- Preparing members for additions and losses of members; providing opportunity to talk about addition and loss experience
- Encouraging in-depth exploration of the topic area

Termination Phase. The usual interventions of this phase include:

- Being sure members know the termination date in advance
- Providing adequate time in as many sessions as necessary to work through feelings about separation (anger, sadness, joy, indifference, etc.)
- Helping members leave with positive feelings by identifying positive changes that have occurred in individual members and in the group as a whole
- Exploring the support systems available to individual members and bridging the gap where possible (to another agency, another therapist, a community support group, etc.)
- Maintaining a focus on resolving the loss

Therapeutic Groups

There are several different types of groups that are therapeutic support groups, but not group therapy.

Self-Help Groups. The major operating principle in self-help groups is that the help given to members comes from the members themselves. The role of the nurse in self-help groups is that of a resource person. There is a wide variety of self-help groups available in this and other countries. Some are:

- Recovery Incorporated, and Schizophrenics Anonymous (concerned with mental disorder)
- Alcoholics Anonymous, and Narcotics Anonymous (concerned with substance abuse)
- Al-Anon, and Al-a-Teen (concerned with the families of substance abusers)
- Gamblers Anonymous and Gam-Anon (concerned with compulsive gambling)
- Child Abuse Listening Mediation (CALM) and Parents Anonymous (concerned with child abuse)

There are also groups for persons addicted to tobacco; for women who breast feed; for people who are divorced, widowed, or single; for parents of runaways and troubled adolescents; for recently bereaved persons, and others.

Psychoeducation Groups. Psychoeducation groups have the sharing of mental health care information as a primary goal.

They also have the secondary benefit of facilitating the discussion of feelings such as isolation, helplessness, sadness, stigmatization, and/or anger, and possible strategies for dealing with these feelings. Some examples of psychoeducation groups are:

- Medication teaching groups that educate clients and their families about medications, their side effects, the nature and course of their mental disorder, the possibility of relapse without continued drug treatment, and the positive effects medications have on their lives
- Social skills training groups (social skills training is discussed earlier) that coach clients in simple, yet essential, social interactions
- Groups of medically ill clients and their families that focus on the stresses associated with illness and have as their goal the reduction of stress

Activity Therapy Groups.   Activity therapies are manual, recreational, and creative techniques to facilitate personal experiences and increase social responses and self-esteem. Nurses often lead creative arts therapy groups or use their principles to reach beyond the ordinary realm of verbal communication with clients in the following ways:

- Poetry therapy groups, helping members get in touch with feelings and emotions through reading poetry or possibly writing poetry themselves.
- Art therapy groups, in which art produced during the session is used as the basis for discussion and for exploring members' feelings,
- Music therapy groups, consisting of singing, rhythm, body movement, and listening, and designed to increase members' concentration, memory retention, conceptual development, rhythmic development, movement behavior, verbal and nonverbal retention, and expression and discussion of affect.
- Dance therapy groups, for members who find it easier to express nonverbally the feelings and emotions that have been difficult to realize and communicate by other means.
- Bibliotherapy groups, for stimulating group members to compare events and characters in books with their own interpersonal and intrapsychic experiences.

Storytelling Groups.   In storytelling groups, members create a story together, often based on a question by the leader ("What would you title your biography?", or "What would you do if you won the lottery?"), thus stimulating interaction and imagination. Story-telling can help members talk about feelings and connect with one another. It can assist elders in reminiscence work. In addition, sto-rytelling can be fun, generate laughter (and endorphins), and re-duce stress, no matter the client's age.

Family Therapy

In general, family therapists believe that the emotional symptoms or problems of an individual are an expression of emotional symp-toms or problems in a family and/or that the interactions among family members influence the course of a mental disorder. There-fore, family therapists view the family system as a unit of treat-ment. Nurse family therapists should be clinical specialists or advanced practitioners prepared in graduate programs that pro-vide both theory and supervised clinical practice in this specialized area.

Most family therapists recommend that all people in the family constellation participate in the assessment phase of family ther-apy. Different coalitions or subsets may be seen together at differ-ent times to accomplish specific goals. For example, mates are often seen together for the first few sessions. Children four years of age and younger are often not included in ongoing family ther-apy sessions. Some therapists, however, make it a point to bring all the children into therapy for at least two sessions to see how the family operates as a whole.

There are two basic forms of family therapy—insight-oriented and behavioral-oriented—into which all schools of family therapy fit. Some examples of insight-oriented family therapy approaches are:

- Psychodynamic: based on the belief that problems arise be-cause of developmental delays, or current interactions or stresses
- Family of origin therapy: in which the goal is to foster differenti-ation among the members and decrease emotional reactivity

Some examples of behavioral-oriented family therapy approaches are:

- Structural: in which the focus is on systems, subsystems, and boundaries

- Strategic: based on the belief that problems arise because of inequality of power, flawed communication, and repetitive and maladaptive family interaction patterns
- Cognitive-behavioral: based on the belief that problems arise because of how families think and learn

Orientation Phase.   The orientation phase of family therapy focuses on negotiating the contract for treatment and includes the following interventions:

- Assessing the family needs and problems
- Identifying what each member would like changed in the family
- Negotiating a set of attainable goals that everyone is willing to work on
- Facilitating compromise in order to achieve the working goals
- Identifying the means—tasks, strategies, and so on—that will be used to reach the negotiated goals
- Identifying the roles and responsibilities in therapy of the family members and the family therapist

Working Phase.   Therapy for a family system involves understanding and using the here-and-now and understanding the basic processes that occur in families. The following are common interventions used in the working phase:

- Creating a safe setting in which family members can risk looking at themselves and their actions
- Teaching family members how to share their observations with one another
- Asking for, and giving, information in a matter-of-fact, nonjudgmental, congruent way
- Responding as a role model whose meaning or intent can be checked on without fear
- Setting rules for interaction to ensure that all family members participate (e.g., interruptions, acting out, or making it impossible to converse are not tolerated; no one speaks for anyone else)
- Clarifying the content and relationship aspects of messages
- Pointing out significant discrepancies, incongruities, or double-level messages
- Helping everyone speak out clearly so that each can be heard

- Viewing the family as a system and not taking sides
- Showing that anger, pain, and the "forbidden" are safe to look at
- Reeducating family members to be accountable
- Delineating family roles and functions and teaching explicitly about role responses and role choices

Termination Phase. Termination in family therapy is geared toward helping families achieve realistic goals, thus ending therapy with a feeling of accomplishment as a family unit. Family therapy should end when family members can:

- See how they appear to others
- Give feedback to others, telling them how they appear
- Share their hopes, fears, and expectations with one another
- Openly discuss problems with one another
- Openly disagree with one another when appropriate
- Give clear messages
- Check meaning with one another
- Ask for clarification
- Support one another

Cognitive and Behavioral Therapies

Cognitive (thought) and behavioral (action) therapies focus on how an individual thinks and/or learns and how the individual can make changes in thinking by substituting for and displacing disturbing and negative thoughts, or retraining, or learning new ways of behavior. Examples of cognitive therapies are positive imagery, mastery imagery, negative imagery, and attribution restructuring. Examples of behavioral therapies are classical conditioning, operant conditioning, rational emotive therapy, behavior modification, and thought stopping. Dialectical behavioral therapy is an example of a cognitive–behavioral therapy that combines features of both cognitive and behavioral therapies.

The principles of cognitive functioning and behavior typically include:

- What people think affects how they feel.
- What people think is often based upon thinking habits.
- When thinking changes there can be change in feelings.

- People do things when they are rewarded in a way that is meaningful for them, or when something they don't like is removed.

- People don't do things when they get punished, or when something they like is taken away from them.

Positive Imagery.   Positive imagery consists of thinking in a positive way about how an event or experience will unfold. When directed toward an upcoming event, positive imagery serves as a cognitive rehearsal. That is, positive thinking in advance about how a set of behaviors or an event will occur helps the individual to perform more competently in a variety of situations and with an array of appropriate skills.

Mastery Imagery.   Mastery imagery shapes the individual's thoughts about being in control or having mastery over a particular situation. The point is to practice imagined successful behavior change.

Negative Imagery.   Negative imagery is the envisioning of negative events and outcomes. The steps include:

1. Identifying currently held imagery
2. Recognizing the real impact of the behavior
3. Substituting a negative imagery for the currently held imagery

The client is taught to identify the imagery invoked (the thoughts) when beginning a maladaptive behavior, such as substance use. For example, substituting positive imagery, such as "I am so much more relaxed when I use this stuff" with negative imagery, such as "If I use cocaine, I will lose control of my thoughts and feelings. It will cost a lot of money, which I don't have, and will put a larger emotional and physical gap between me and my spouse." Replacing positive imagery with negative imagery, and repeating the negative imagery, are the key components to the effective use of this technique.

Attribution Restructuring.   We label or assign a certain meaning to a circumstance or a set of circumstances (such as expecting a grade of B in a course of study). Then, we attribute associated features or characteristics to that circumstance (being a good student or knowing the course material). Next, we expect a certain outcome based on our attributions, and behave consistently with that explanation. Attribution restructuring involves identifying maladaptive automatic thoughts and attributions and then altering or restructuring the meaning associated with the people, places, things, or other elements of the circumstance or set of circumstances.

Classical Conditioning. Conditioning is learning that occurs through reinforcement. People learn to associate a specific feeling (love) with a specific circumstance (a lover's gentle touch). The circumstance (touch) becomes a conditioned stimulus for the feeling (love). Over time, this association is strengthened through repetition and rehearsal. Learning occurs through reinforcement in which desired behaviors are rewarded and thus persist, and undesired behaviors are punished and thus stopped.

Operant Conditioning. Operant conditioning is based upon the ideas that:

- People are positively reinforced for certain behaviors
- People learn to seek further positive reinforcement by increasing that behavior, and
- Positive reinforcement results from either gaining something desirable, or avoiding something unpleasant

The goal in operant conditioning is to help the individual increase positive reinforcement through more adaptive and efficient behavior.

Rational Emotive Therapy. Rational emotive therapy (RET) emphasizes the cognitive causes of emotional problems and the need for the individual to take personal responsibility for substituting more rational personal life philosophies and attitudes based on accurate and correctly perceived realities for health-damaging thought habits and irrational beliefs (those that lack sound reason and judgment). An example of an irrational thought is: "I should always be capable, successful, and on top of things (if I'm not, I'm an inadequate, incompetent, hopeless failure)." Because RET focuses on a logical perspective of problems, it has an appealing and manageable therapeutic style to which many adults can relate.

Behavior Modification

Behavior modification focuses on a target behavior that has become problematic for the individual (e.g., overeating) or for the community (e.g., loud, verbal outbursts). The behavior is observed and tracked in objective and measurable terms, then addressed with a behavior modification plan.

Desensitization.   Desensitization is another behavioral modification regimen. Therapist and client together develop a hierarchy of behaviors that are ordered according to how distressing they are for the individual. The client imagines being in certain situations at various levels of distress (e.g., a client with a fear of flying might develop a hierarchy that progresses from seeing an airplane in the distance to flying in one) and learns to cope with the anxiety engendered by each step before moving on to the next higher level of distress. The final steps of the desensitization process include encouraging the client to try some of these behaviors in real life, after the simulations have been successful.

Thought Stopping.   The technique of thought stopping focuses on helping a person to stop negative or maladaptive thinking by imagining an image, a sensation, or a circumstance associated with halting a particular thought process. This might include visualizing a traffic stop sign, imagining hearing the word "stop" said loudly, or imagining the tactile sensation of leaning against a closed door. The individual uses these techniques whenever the identified negative or maladaptive thought occurs. Over time, stopping these thoughts almost becomes automatic.

Dialectical Behavioral Therapy.   Dialectical behavioral therapy (DBT) was specifically developed for the outpatient treatment of chronically suicidal persons with borderline personality disorder. DBT teaches clients four skills in a clearly structured format:

1. mindfulness (attention to one's experience)
2. interpersonal effectiveness
3. emotional regulation, and
4. distress tolerance

This concept of therapy is based on the necessity of accepting maladaptive behavior patterns (a cognitive feature) while working to change it (the behavioral feature).

Crisis Intervention

A crisis is an acute, time-limited state of disequilibrium resulting from situational, developmental, or societal sources of stress. An individual is in a state of crisis when usual problem-solving or adapting methods are inadequate to resolve a problem or conflict. Crisis situations are also turning points or junctures in a person's life that result in a new equilibrium. The new equilibrium may be close to that of the precrisis state, or it may be a more positive or more negative state. If the new equilibrium is more positive, the person experiences personal growth, increased competence, a better social network, newfound problem-solving abilities, or an improved self-image. If the new equilibrium is more negative, it is possible that the individual may lose skills, regress, develop socially unacceptable behaviors, or develop a mental disorder.

A person experiencing a crisis alone is more vulnerable to unsuccessful negotiation than a person working through a crisis with help. The therapeutic approach that helps a person to negotiate a crisis is called crisis intervention—short-term action-oriented assistance focused on problem-solving, with a goal of restoring the individual's equilibrium. This is why crisis intervention is sometimes referred to as primary prevention for posttraumatic stress disorder (PTSD).

Types of Crises. A crisis can be situational, resulting from three sources: material or environmental (e.g., fire or natural disaster); personal or physical (e.g., heart attack, diagnosis of fatal illness, bodily disfigurement); and interpersonal or social (e.g., death of a loved one or divorce). A crisis can be maturational, involving life cycle changes or normal transitions of human development (e.g., puberty, marriage, middle age, retirement).

Balancing Factors. Three balancing factors are important to the successful resolution of the disequilibrium caused by crisis:

1. Perception of the event: how individuals perceive and understand the event/crisis in their lives.
2. Situational supports: the availability of people who can help individuals in crisis solve the problem.
3. Coping mechanisms: the coping repertoire the individual has used with success in the past (Aguilera, 1998).

Stages of Crisis Intervention. Roberts' seven-stage model of crisis intervention (2000) has been used to help people in crisis. The seven stages that should undergird any plan of care for a client in crisis are:

1. Plan and conduct a thorough assessment (including suicide lethality assessment, assessment of dangerousness to self or others, and assessment of immediate psychosocial needs).
2. Make interpersonal contact, establish rapport, and rapidly establish the relationship (conveying genuine regard and respect for the client, acceptance, reassurance, and a nonjudgmental attitude).

3. Examine the dimensions of the problem in order to define it (including the "last straw" of the precipitating event).

4. Encourage an exploration of feelings and emotions (through active listening).

5. Explore and assess past coping attempts and generate and explore alternatives and previously untried coping methods or solutions.

6. Restore cognitive functioning through the implementation of an action plan based on cognitive mastery.

7. Follow up with the client and leave the door open for future contact, especially around the time of the anniversary of the event (exactly one month or one year after the victimization).

Types of Crisis Intervention. Several different modalities can be used to implement the guidelines above.

- Crisis counseling, a type of brief, solution-focused therapy that lasts for five or six sessions

- Telephone counseling through hotlines available around the clock, staffed by volunteers who have professional consultation available to them

- Taking steps to provide shelter for a homeless person, a safe house for an abused woman and her children, or arranging for in-home health care

- Providing anticipatory guidance in anticipation of the potential for crisis, thus averting it (preparing a child and family for a tonsillectomy, preparing a list of helpful phone numbers for the newly discharged client with schizophrenia, discussing methods of contraception with sexually active persons)

- Helping develop social supports (introducing a woman whose husband is an alcoholic to Al-Anon; giving a rape victim the telephone number of the rape crisis hotline; referring a family with a terminally ill member to a local hospice)

- Critical incident stress debriefing, a seven-phase group meeting with both psychologic and psychoeducation elements, that offers individuals affected by a traumatic event the opportunity to share their thoughts and feelings in a safe and controlled environment

- Home crisis visits, when telephone counseling does not suffice or when there is a need to obtain additional information by direct observation

- Community-based programs such as mobile crisis units, designed to deliver crisis services to any location in the community without delay

- Disaster assistance that meets acute needs at the disaster site (food, shelter, medical care) and the psychologic needs of victims both during and after the disaster

Complementary and Alternative Therapies

Alternative therapy is an umbrella term for hundreds of therapies drawn from all over the world. Many forms have been handed down over thousands of years, both orally and as written records. These are based on the medical systems of ancient peoples, including Egyptians, Chinese, Asian Indians, Greeks, and Native Peoples. Others, such as osteopathy and chiropractic, have evolved in the United States over the past two centuries. Still others, such as some of the mind–body and bioelectromagnetic approaches, are on the frontier of scientific knowledge and understanding.

Studies show that more than one-third of Americans use alternative treatments in a given year. Among people with mental disorders, the use is even more common. Many individuals with anxiety attacks (43 percent) and adults with severe depression (41 percent) utilize alternative therapies. Most of them also continue to use conventional health care (Kessler, Walters, & Forthofer, 2001).

Nursing is in a unique position to take a leadership role in integrating alternative healing methods into Western health care systems. Historically, we have used our hands, heart, and head in more natural and traditional healing interactions. As nurses, by virtue of our education and relationships with clients, we can help consumers assert their right to choose their own healing journey and the quality of their life and death experiences (Fontaine, 2000).

Acupuncture.   Acupuncture, acupressure, Jin Shin Jyutsu, Jin Shin Do, and reflexology are different forms of the same practice of stimulating points on the body to balance the body's life energy. Frequently these practices are part of a holistic approach to wellness and are combined with diet, herbs, mind–body techniques, and spiritual therapies.

When the flow of energy becomes blocked or congested, people experience discomfort or pain on a physical level, may feel frustrated or irritable on an emotional level, and may experience a sense of vulnerability or lack of purpose in life on a spiritual level. The goal of care is to recognize and manage the disruption before illness or disease occurs. Pressure point practitioners bring balance to the body's energies, which promotes optimal health and well-being, and facilitates people's own healing capacity.

Animal-Assisted Therapy. Animal-assisted therapy is the use of specifically selected animals as a treatment modality in health and human service settings. Accredited professionals guide the human–animal interaction toward specific, individualized therapeutic goals. A variety of goals can be addressed: cognitive goals such as improved memory or verbal expression; emotional goals such as increased self-esteem and motivation; social goals such as building rapport and improved socialization skills; and physical goals such as balance and mobility.

For many people, interacting with a pet is less stressful than interacting with other people. In comparison to people, animals are nonjudgmental and accepting. This unconditional support system can be accessed at any time of day or night when one lives with a pet. Loneliness, lack of companionship, and lack of social support are major risk factors for depression and suicide, which can be offset by the presence of a loved pet. Animals also facilitate socializing within the neighborhood by getting owners out of the house and providing a topic of conversation. Even sitting and looking at fish in an aquarium relaxes and relieves anxiety for many people. Children with short attention spans are able to sustain attention longer when interacting with animals (Hart, 2000).

Aromatherapy. Aromatherapy is the therapeutic use of essential oils in which the odor or fragrance plays an important part. It is an offshoot of herbal medicine, with the basis of action the same as that of modern pharmacology. The chemicals found in the essential oils are absorbed into the body, resulting in physiological or psychological benefit. Essential oils are extracted from plants and are massaged into the skin, inhaled, placed in baths, used as compresses, or mixed into ointments. Different oils may calm, stimulate, improve sleep, change eating habits, or boost the immune system. Some oils cause the brain to release enkephalins, which decrease the perception of pain and increase the sense of well-being (Ratey, 2001). Oils you will find used in the mental health field include:

- **Anxiety:** basil, bergamot, chamomile, green apple, lemon balm, neroli, and orange
- **Depression:** bergamot, geranium, jasmine, lemon balm, rose, and ylang ylang

- **Insomnia:** chamomile, clary sage, lavender, marjoram, neroli, and vetiver
- **Memory/mental function:** basil, ginger, rosemary, thyme
- **Alertness:** peppermint

Essential oils are quite potent and can irritate the skin, so they should be diluted with a carrier oil before being used on the skin. Carrier oils contain vitamins, proteins, and minerals that provide added nutrients to the body. Carrier oils include apricot kernel oil, sunflower oil, soy oil, sweet almond oil, grapeseed oil, sesame oil, avocado oil, jojoba, and wheat-germ oil.

Ayurveda.   The Indian system of medicine, Ayurveda, is at least 2,500 years old. Illness is viewed as a state of imbalance among the body's systems. Ayurveda emphasizes the interdependence of the health of the individual and the quality of societal life. Mentally healthy people have good memory, comprehension, intelligence, and reasoning ability. Emotionally healthy people experience evenly balanced emotional states and a sense of well-being or happiness. Physically healthy people have abundant energy with proper functioning of the senses, digestion, and elimination. From a spiritual perspective, healthy people have a sense of aliveness and richness of life, are developing in the direction of their full potential, and are in a good relationship with themselves, other people, and the larger cosmos.

Nutritional counseling, massage, natural medicines, meditations, yoga, and other modalities are used to treat many disorders. This ancient system has adapted to modern science and technology, including biomedical science and quantum physics.

Traditional Chinese Medicine.   Traditional Chinese Medicine has developed over 3,000 years and seeks to balance the flow of *qi* (chee), the energy or life force of a person. In traditional Chinese medicine the mind, body, spirit, and emotions are never separated. Practitioners are trained to use a variety of ancient and modern therapeutic methods, including acupuncture, herbal medicine, massage, heat therapy, Qi Gong, Tai Chi, and nutritional and lifestyle counseling.

Chiropractic.   Chiropractic is the third largest independent health profession in the Western world after conventional medicine and dentistry. It is based on the premise that the spine is literally the backbone of human health. Misalignments of the vertebrae or loss of mobility in the facet joints caused by poor posture or trauma result in pressure on the spinal cord, which may lead to diminished function and illness. Three primary clinical goals guide chiropractic intervention: (1) reduce or eliminate pain; (2) correct the spinal dysfunction; and (3) use preventive maintenance to assure the problem does not recur.

Curanderismo. Curanderismo is a cultural healing tradition found in Latin American countries and among many Latinos in the United States. Although it is a traditional healing system, it utilizes Western biomedical beliefs, treatments, and practices. Three levels of care are practiced among curanderos and curanderas. These three levels are (1) the material level, (2) the spiritual level, and (3) the mental level. Healers have the gift for working at only one of these levels. Healers working at the mental level have the ability to transmit, channel, and focus mental vibrations in a way that directly affects a person's mental or physical condition. When working with mental conditions, they send vibrations into the person's mind to manipulate energies and modify behavior.

Herbal Medicine. Herbal medicine is used by 80 percent of the world's population. Even though only a tiny fraction of plants have been studied for medicinal benefits, plant-derived products are used regularly by conventional health care providers. Twenty-five percent of all prescription drugs sold in the United States is derived from plants. Because herbs are marketed as "natural" or promoted as foods, consumers may assume incorrectly that herbs are safe and without side effects. It is important that you remember that natural remedies be approached with respect and that you teach people that although herbs are generally much safer than prescription drugs, if abused or overused they can cause harm.

Herbs you will find used in the mental health field include:

- **Anxiety:** chamomile
- **Depression:** St. John's wort and SAMe
- **Mood swings:** ginseng
- **Insomnia:** catnip, hops, lemon balm, melatonin, passion flower, or valerian
- **Memory:** ginkgo
- **Alcohol or drug withdrawal:** chamomile, evening primrose oil, ginseng, and valerian

Herbs are drugs and you need to treat them with respect. The vast majority of herbal medicines present no danger. Some can, however, cause serious side effects if taken in excess or, for some, if taken over a prolonged period of time. Herbs can also interact with drugs and caution should be used when combining herbs with prescription and OTC medications. For example St. John's wort should not be combined with antidepressants, as their effects may increase. St. John's wort reduces the effectiveness of birth control pills, HIV treatment medications, and the asthma medication theophylline. It is important that people investigate herb–drug interactions before using herbs as an alternative therapy.

Hypnotherapy and Guided Imagery.   Hypnosis and guided imagery are states of attentive and focused concentration during which people are highly responsive to suggestion. Therapists help people learn methods to take advantage of the mind/body/spirit connection through the medium of relaxation and imagination. Hypnosis and imagery cannot make people do anything against their will. These therapies can be used to help people gain self-control, improve self-esteem, and become more autonomous. People who are imprisoned by negative beliefs see themselves as hopeless, helpless victims. With hypnosis or guided imagery, they can learn how to substitute positive, empowering messages. These procedures are unsuitable for people with active psychosis or somatic delusions. It is generally considered that these individuals are often bombarded with too many images already, and are unable to differentiate between voluntary and involuntary images.

Massage Therapy.   Massage therapy, the scientific manipulation of the soft tissues of the body, is a healing art, an act of physical caring, and a way of communicating without words. The goal of massage therapy is to achieve or increase health and well-being and to help people heal themselves. On the mental level massage therapy induces a relaxed state of alertness, reduces mental stress, thus clearing the mind, and increases one's capacity for clearer thinking. On the emotional level massage therapy satisfies the need for caring and nurturing touch, increases feelings of well-being, decreases mild depression, enhances self-image, reduces levels of anxiety, and increases awareness of the mind–body connection.

Meditation.   Meditation is a general term for a wide range of practices that involve relaxing the body and stilling the mind. Meditation is a process that anyone can use to calm down, cope with stress, and, for those with spiritual inclinations, feel as one with God or the universe. Meditation can be practiced individually or in groups and is easy to learn. It requires no change in belief system and is compatible with most religious practices. People who meditate say that they have clearer minds and sharper thoughts. The brain seems to clear itself so that new ideas and beliefs become available. This clearer mind may be accompanied by a cognitive restructuring in which people interpret life events in a more positive, more realistic fashion. Meditation's residual effects—improved stress-coping abilities—are a protection against daily stress and anxiety.

Native American Healing.   Spirituality and medicine are inseparable in Native American tradition. Medicine women and men see themselves as channels through which the Great Power helps others achieve well-being in mind, body, and spirit. The only healer is the One who created all things. Medicine people consider that they have certain knowledge to put things together to help the sick person heal and that knowledge has to be dispensed in a certain way, often through ritual or ceremony. The healer enters into the healing relationship with love and compassion. The two individuals experience a joining or merging as this process unfolds. This merger symbolizes the cementing of people with the Divine Spirit.

Health is viewed as a balance or harmony of mind and body. The goal is to be in harmony with all things, which means first being in harmony with oneself. It is believed that most illness begins in the head and people must get rid of ideas, which predispose illness. If the mind is negative, the body will be drained, making it more vulnerable. When people open up to the universe, learn what is good for them, and find ways to be happier, they can begin to work toward a longer and healthier life.

Prayer.   Prayer is most often defined simply as a form of communication and fellowship with the Deity or Creator. All cultures have some form of prayer. Life-affirming beliefs and philosophies nourish people. They meditate and say prayers that elicit physiological calm and a sense of peacefulness, both of which contribute to longer survival.

T'ai Chi.   T'ai Chi and Qigong are Chinese practices consisting of breathing and mental exercises combined with body movements. They are easy and nontiring exercises that contain sets of moves designed to gather qi, or energy. Most people spend 30 minutes a day doing the exercises and another 30 minutes in meditation. Practitioners discover how to generate more energy and conserve what they have in order to maintain health or treat illness. The benefits of T'ai Chi are seen in conditions such as hypertension, osteoporosis, and arthritis. T'ai Chi can decrease stress and fatigue, improve mood, and increase energy. It is especially helpful in improving balance in older adults, which decreases the risk of falls.

Therapeutic Touch.   Popularized by nursing professor Dolores Krieger in the 1970s, therapeutic touch is practiced by registered nurses and others to relieve pain and stress. It is believed that people must, and do, heal themselves. Healing environments are created when nurses enter into caring moments with clients in which the nurse becomes a resource for clients to self-heal. The nurse assesses where the person's energy field is weak or congested and then uses her/his hands to direct energy into the field to balance it. Indications include irritability and anxiety; lethargy, fatigue, and depression; premenstrual syndrome; nausea and vomiting, chemotherapy and radiation sickness; wound and bone healing; and acute musculoskeletal problems such as sprains and muscle spasms. Therapeutic touch produces a sense of well-being and relaxation for both the nurse and the client.

Yoga.   Yoga has been practiced for thousands of years in India, where it is a way of life that includes ethical models for behavior and mental and physical exercises aimed at producing spiritual enlightenment. It is a method for life that can complement and enhance any system of religion, or it can be practiced completely apart from religion. The Western approach to yoga tends to be more fitness oriented, with the goals of managing stress, learning to relax, and increasing vitality and well-being. A typical yoga session lasts 20 minutes to an hour. Some spend 30 minutes doing the poses and another 30 minutes doing breathing practices and meditations. Others spend the majority of the time doing poses and end with a short meditation or relaxation procedure. Even for those who are stiff and out of shape, sick, or weak, sets of easy exercises can help to loosen the joints and stimulate circulation. If practiced regularly, these simple exercises alone make a great difference in people's health and well-being.

Nursing and alternative therapies share the focus on what is unique about the individual and her/his role in healing. The individual is always at the center of treatment interventions with the emphasis on growth toward health. Health promotion is a lifelong process that focuses on optimal development of our physical, emotional, mental, and spiritual selves.

MEDICATIONS

Several of the most commonly used medications in the specialty area of psychiatry are listed here. The psychiatric medications covered are listed alphabetically by generic name. The index includes the generic and the brand names of these medications. When a medication treats a nonpsychiatric condition as well as psychiatric disorders (such as valproic acid for mania), the psychiatric dosing and information is accentuated. The source of this information is Wilson, B. A., Shannon, M. T., & Stang, C. L. (2003). *Nurse's Drug Guide 2003.* Upper Saddle River, New Jersey: Prentice Hall.

ALPRAZOLAM (al-pray'zoe-lam)
Trade name: Xanax
Classifications: CNS AGENT; BENZODIAZEPINE ANXIOLYTIC; SEDATIVE-HYPNOTIC
Pregnancy category: D
Controlled substance: Schedule IV

ACTIONS/PHARMACODYNAMICS CNS depressant. Mode of action not known but appears to act at the limbic, thalamic, and hypothalamic levels of the CNS. It is associated with significantly less drowsiness. Has antidepressant as well as anxiolytic actions.

USES Management of anxiety disorders or for short-term relief of anxiety symptoms. Also used as adjunct in management of anxiety associated with depression and agitation and for panic disorders, such as agoraphobia.

ROUTE & DOSAGE
Anxiety Disorders
Adult: 0.25–0.5 mg t.i.d. (max 4 mg/d).
Geriatric: 0.125-0.25 mg b.i.d.
Panic Attacks
Adult: 1–2 mg t.i.d. (max * mg/d).

PHARMACOKINETICS
Absorption: rapidly absorbed.
Peak: 1–2 h.
Distribution: crosses placenta.
Metabolism: oxidized in liver to inactive metabolites.
Elimination: half-life 12–15 h; renal elimination.

Common side effects are shown in *italic,* life-threatening effects are underlined, generic names are in **bold,** and drug classes are in SMALL CAPS.

CONTRAINDICATIONS & PRECAUTIONS Contraindicated in: sensitivity to benzodiazepines; acute narrow angle glaucoma; pulmonary disease; use alone in primary depression or psychotic disorders; during pregnancy (category D), in nursing mothers and children <18 y.
Cautious use in: impaired renal or hepatic function; history of alcoholism; geriatric and debilitated clients. Effectiveness for long-term treatment (>4 mo) not established.

ADVERSE/SIDE EFFECTS CNS: *drowsiness, sedation,* light-headedness, dizziness, syncope, depression, headache, confusion, insomnia, nervousness, fatigue, clumsiness, unsteadiness, rigidity, tremor, restlessness, paradoxical excitement, hallucinations. **CV:** tachycardia, hypotension, ECG changes. **Other:** blurred vision, dyspnea.

DRUG INTERACTIONS Alcohol and other CNS DEPRESSANTS, ANTICONVULSANTS, ANTIHISTAMINES, BARBITURATES, NARCOTIC ANALGESICS, BENZODIAZEPINES compound CNS depressant effects; **cimetidine, disulfiram** increase **alprazolam** effects (decreased metabolism); oral contraceptives may increase or decrease **alprazolam** effects.

NURSING IMPLICATIONS

Administration

- **Alprazolam** may be administered without regard to meals.
- Store in light-resistant containers at 15–30C (59–86F), unless otherwise directed.

Assessment & Intervention

- Clients receiving continuing therapy should have periodic blood counts, urinalyses, and blood chemistry studies.
- Drowsiness and sedation are the most common side effects. Monitor especially the elderly or debilitated, who may require supervised ambulation or side rails.

Client & Family Education

- Adverse reactions, which may occur during early high-dose therapy, usually disappear with continuing therapy. Advise client to keep prescriber informed; dosage adjustments may be indicated. Instruct client to make position changes slowly and in stages.
- **Alprazolam** potentiates effects of alcohol **(ETOH)** and other central nervous system (CNS) depressants; caution client not to use them or OTC medications containing antihistamines (sleep aids, cold, hay fever, or allergy remedies) without consulting prescriber.

Common side effects are shown in *italic*, life-threatening effects are <u>underlined</u>, generic names are in **bold**, and drug classes are in SMALL CAPS.

- Advise client to avoid driving and other potentially hazardous activities until reaction to drug is determined.
- Following continuous use, dosage should be tapered off before drug is stopped. Abrupt discontinuation of drug may cause withdrawal symptoms: nausea, vomiting, abdominal and muscle cramps, sweating, confusion, tremors, convulsions.

AMITRIPTYLINE (a-mee-trip′ti-leen)
Trade names: Amitril, Apo-Amitriptyline (Canada), Elavil, Emitrip, Endep, Enovil, Levate (Canada), Meravil, Novotriptyn (Canada)
Classifications: CNS AGENT; PSYCHOTHERAPEUTIC; TRICYCLIC ANTIDE-PRESSANT
Pregnancy category: C

ACTIONS/PHARMACODYNAMICS Among the most active of the tricyclic antidepressants (TCAs) in inhibition of serotonin uptake from synaptic gap; also inhibits norepinephrine reuptake to a moderate degree. Restoration of the levels of these neurotransmitters is a proposed mechanism of antidepressant action. Has H2-receptor blocking activity (inhibits gastric acid secretion) and prominent anticholinergic and sedative actions.

USES Depression. Off label uses: prophylaxis for cluster, migraine, and chronic tension headaches; intractable pain, peptic ulcer disease, to increase muscle strength in myotonic dystrophy, to treat pathologic weeping and laughing secondary to forebrain disease, for eating disorders associated with depression (anorexia or bulimia), and as sedative for nondepressed clients.

ROUTE & DOSAGE
Antidepressant
Adult: 75–100 mg/d; may gradually increase to 150–300 mg/d (use lower doses in outpatients). IM 20–30 mg q.i.d. until client can take PO.
Geriatric: 10–25 mg h.s., may gradually increase to 25–150 mg/d.
Adolescent: 10 mg t.i.d. and 20 mg h.s.

PHARMACOKINETICS
Absorption: rapidly absorbed from GI and injection sites.
Peak levels: 2–12 h.
Distribution: crosses placenta.

Common side effects are shown in *italic,* life-threatening effects are <u>underlined</u>, generic names are in **bold,** and drug classes are in SMALL CAPS.

Metabolism: metabolized in liver to active metabolite.
Elimination: half-life 10–50 h; primarily excreted in urine; enters breast milk.

CONTRAINDICATIONS & PRECAUTIONS

Contraindicated in: acute recovery period after MI, history of seizure disorders, pregnancy (category C), nursing mothers, children under 12 y.
Cautious use in: prostatic hypertrophy, history of urinary retention or obstruction; angle-closure glaucoma; diabetes mellitus; hyperthyroidism; client with cardiovascular, hepatic, or renal dysfunction; client with suicidal tendency, electroshock therapy; elective surgery; schizophrenia; respiratory disorders; elderly, adolescents.

ADVERSE/SIDE EFFECTS CNS: *drowsiness, sedation, dizziness,* nervousness, restlessness, fatigue, headache, insomnia, abnormal movements (extrapyramidal symptoms), seizures. **CV**: *orthostatic hypotension,* tachycardia, palpitation, ECG changes. **Eye**: blurred vision, mydriasis. **GI**: *dry mouth,* increased appetite especially for sweets, *constipation,* weight gain, sour or metallic taste, nausea, vomiting. **Other**: *urinary retention,* <u>bone marrow depression</u> (rare).

DRUG INTERACTIONS ANTIHYPERTENSIVES may increase some antihypertensive response; CNS DEPRESSANTS, alcohol, HYPNOTICS, BARBITURATES, SEDATIVES potentiate CNS depression; ANTICOAGULANTS, ORAL, may increase hypoprothombinemic effect; **ethchlorvynol,** transient delirium; **levodopa,** SYMPATHOMIMETICS (e.g., epinephrine, norepinephrine), possibility of sympathetic hyperactivity with hypertension and hyperpyrexia; MAO INHIBITORS, possibility of severe reactions, toxic psychosis, cardiovascular instability; **methylphenidate** increases plasma TCA levels; THYROID DRUGS may increase possibility of arrhythmias; **cimetidine** may increase plasma TCA levels.

NURSING IMPLICATIONS

Administration

- Oral drug may be taken with or immediately after food to reduce possibility of GI irritation. Tablet may be crushed if client is unwilling to take it whole; administer with food or fluid.
- Dose increases by 25–50 mg are preferably made in late afternoon or at bedtime because sedative action precedes antidepressant effect.

Common side effects are shown in *italic,* life-threatening effects are <u>underlined,</u> generic names are in **bold,** and drug classes are in SMALL CAPS.

- A single dose at bedtime is useful to promote sleep or for clients who complain of dizziness or when daytime sedation interferes with work productivity. Drug effect on depression is not affected by time of day dose is taken.
- Maintenance regimen is usually continued for at least 3 mo to prevent relapse. Typical length of therapy for depression is 6 mo–1 y.
- Abrupt discontinuation of therapy can precipitate withdrawal symptoms (headache, nausea, malaise, musculoskeletal pain, panic attack, weakness). This reaction can be avoided by tapering dosage over 2 wk.
- Store drug at 15–30C (59–86F) unless otherwise directed by manufacturer. Protect from light.

Assessment & Intervention

- Baseline and periodic leukocyte and differential counts, BP, cardiac, renal, and hepatic function tests, and eye examinations (including glaucoma testing) are recommended particularly for the elderly, adolescents, and for clients receiving high doses or prolonged therapy.
- Monitor BP and pulse rate in clients with preexisting cardiovascular disease. Withhold drug if there is a rise or fall in systolic BP (by 10–20 mm Hg), or a sudden increase or a significant change in pulse rate or rhythm. Notify health care provider.
- Monitor I&O, including bowel elimination pattern.
- During initial therapy, be alert to drowsiness and dizziness. Institute measures to prevent falling.
- If a client uses excessive amounts of alcohol, it should be borne in mind that the potentiation of **amitriptyline** effects may increase the dangers of overdosage or suicide attempt.
- When used for migraine prophylaxis, therapeutic effect may occur in 1–6 wk. Drug is usually discontinued after client has been headache-free for 1–2 mo. If headache recurs, prescriber may prescribe another course of treatment.

Client & Family Education

- Monitor weight. **Amitriptyline** may increase the appetite and cause weight gain; some clients develop a craving for sweets.
- Tolerance or adaptation to distressing anticholinergic actions usually develops after client goes on maintenance regimen. Keep prescriber informed.
- Advise client that dry mouth can be relieved by taking frequent sips of water and by increasing total fluid intake.

Common side effects are shown in *italic,* life-threatening effects are <u>underlined</u>, generic names are in **bold,** and drug classes are in SMALL CAPS.

- Instruct client to change position slowly and in stages. Support stockings may help. Consult health care provider.
- Avoid potentially hazardous activities, such as driving, until response to the drug is known.
- Desired therapeutic effects for depression may not be evident until after 3–4 wk of therapy, because of long serum half-life.
- Advise client not to use OTC drugs while on TCA therapy. Many preparations contain sympathomimetic amines.
- Inform client that **amitriptyline** may make urine blue-green.

BUPROPION (byoo-pro′pi-on)
Trade names: Wellbutrin, Wellbutrin SR, Zyban
Classification: ANTIDEPRESSANT
Pregnancy category: B

ACTIONS/PHARMACODYNAMICS The neurochemical mechanism of **bupropion** is unknown. It does not inhibit monamine oxidase. Compared to tricyclic antidepressants, it is a weak blocker of neural uptake of serotonin and norepinephrine.

USES Indicated for mental depression; since it has been associated with increased risk of seizures, it is not the agent of first choice; adjunct for smoking cessation. Off label uses: cyclic mood disorders, schizoaffective disorders.

ROUTE & DOSAGE
Depression
Adult: 75–100 mg t.i.d.; doses >450 mg/d are associated with an increased risk of adverse reactions (including seizures); max 150 mg/dose; start with 75 mg t.i.d. or 100 mg b.i.d. and increase dose q3d to 300 mg/d.
Geriatric: 50–100 mg/d, may increase by 50–100 mg q3–4d.
Smoking Cessation
Adult: start with 150 mg q.d. × 3 d, then increase to 150 mg b.i.d. (max 300 mg/d) for 7–12 wk.

PHARMACOKINETICS
Absorption: readily absorbed from GI tract.
Onset: 3–4 wk.
Peak: 1–3 h.
Metabolism: metabolized in liver (including first pass metabolism) to active metabolites.

Elimination: half-life 8–24 h; 80% excreted in urine as inactive metabolites.

CONTRAINDICATIONS & PRECAUTIONS

Contraindicated in: hypersensitivity to drug, history of seizure disorder, current or prior diagnosis of bulimia or anorexia nervosa, concurrent administration of MAO inhibitor, head trauma, CNS tumor, recent MI, nursing mothers.

Cautious use in: renal or hepatic function impairment, drug abuse or dependence, pregnancy (category B).

ADVERSE/SIDE EFFECTS CNS: *seizures.* The risk of seizure appears to be strongly associated with dose (especially >450 mg/d) and may be increased by predisposing factors (e.g., head trauma, CNS tumor) or a history of prior seizure; *agitation, insomnia, dry mouth, blurred vision, headache, dizziness, tremor.* **GI:** *nausea, vomiting, constipation.* **CV:** tachycardia. **Other:** weight loss, weight gain, rash.

DRUG INTERACTIONS Bupropion may increase metabolism of **carbamazepine, cimetidine, phenytoin, phenobarbital,** decreasing their effect; may increase incidence of adverse effects of **levodopa,** MAO INHIBITORS.

NURSING IMPLICATIONS

Administration

- **Bupropion** may be administered with meals to decrease the incidence of nausea and vomiting.
- Increases in dosage should not exceed 100 mg/d over a 3 d period. Greater increments increase the seizure potential.
- Store away from heat and direct light as well as moist areas.
- Do not crush the sustained release (SR) or extended release forms of this drug.

Assessment & Intervention

- Use extreme caution when administering drug to client with history of seizures, cranial trauma, or other factors predisposing to seizures.
- During sudden and large increments in dose, seizure potential is increased.
- A substantial proportion of clients experience some degree of increased restlessness, agitation, anxiety, and insomnia. Symptoms may require treatment or discontinuation of drug.

Common side effects are shown in *italic,* life-threatening effects are <u>underlined,</u> generic names are in **bold,** and drug classes are in SMALL CAPS.

- Monitor for delusions, hallucinations, psychotic episodes, confusion, and paranoia.
- **Bupropion** may cause ECG changes such as premature beats and nonspecific ST-T changes with long-term use.
- Hepatic and renal function tests should be monitored while client is on this drug.
- The full antidepressant effect of drug may not be realized for 4 or more weeks.

Client & Family Education

- Drug should be taken at same times each day.
- Weight gain of ≈2 kg (5 lb) may occur.
- Alcohol increases the risk of seizures, in addition to being a depressant. Therefore, its consumption should be minimized or, preferably, avoided.
- Ability to perform tasks requiring judgment or motor and cognitive skills may be impaired. Client should refrain from driving or other hazardous activities until reaction to drug is known.
- Client should check with prescriber before discontinuing this medication. Gradual dosage reduction may be necessary to prevent adverse effects.
- Advise client not to take any OTC drugs without informing health care provider.

BUSPIRONE (byoo-spye'rone)
Trade name: BuSpar
Classifications: CNS AGENT; ANXIOLYTIC
Pregnancy category: B

ACTIONS/PHARMACODYNAMICS Nonbenzodiazepine unrelated to other psychotherapeutic agents. Does not have muscle relaxant or anticonvulsant effects. Abuse potential is minimal. Unlike other anxiolytics, it seems to cause less clinically significant impairment of cognitive and motor performance and produces minimal if any interaction with other brain depressants, including alcohol.

USE Management of anxiety disorders and for short-term treatment of generalized anxiety.

ROUTE & DOSAGE
Anxiety
Adult: 7.5–15 mg in divided doses; may increase by 5 mg/d q2–3d as needed (max 60 mg/d).

Common side effects are shown in *italic,* life-threatening effects are <u>underlined</u>, generic names are in **bold**, and drug classes are in SMALL CAPS.

Geriatric: 5 mg/d; may increase to max 60 mg/d.

PHARMACOKINETICS

Absorption: readily absorbed from GI tract but undergoes first pass metabolism.
Onset: 5–7 d.
Peak: 1 h.
Duration: 6–8 h.
Metabolism: metabolized in the liver.
Elimination: half-life 2–4 h; 30–63% excreted in urine as metabolites within 24 h.

CONTRAINDICATIONS & PRECAUTIONS

Contraindicated in: safe use in pregnancy (category B), lactation, or in children <18 y not established.
Cautious use in: renal or hepatic impairment.

ADVERSE/SIDE EFFECTS CNS: numbness, paresthesia, tremors, *dizziness, headache,* nervousness, *drowsiness,* light-headedness, dream disturbances, decreased concentration, excitement, mood changes. **CV:** tachycardia, palpitation. **Eye:** blurred vision. **GI:** *nausea,* vomiting, dry mouth, abdominal/gastric distress, diarrhea, constipation. **GU:** urinary frequency, hesitancy. **Musculoskeletal:** arthralgias. **Respiratory:** hyperventilation, shortness of breath. **Skin:** rash, edema, pruritus, flushing, easy bruising, hair loss, dry skin. **Other:** fatigue, weakness.

DIAGNOSTIC TEST INTERFERENCE Buspirone may increase serum concentrates of hepatic aminotransferases (ALT, AST).

DRUG INTERACTIONS MAO INHIBITORS, hypertension; **trazodone,** possible increase in liver transaminases; increased **haloperidol** serum levels.

NURSING IMPLICATIONS

Administration

• Administer with food to decrease first-pass metabolism. Rate of absorption may be delayed, but administration with food increases bioavailability of drug.

Assessment & Intervention

• **Buspirone** may displace **digoxin** from its serum binding. This could increase the potential for toxic serum levels of digoxin.

Common side effects are shown in *italic,* life-threatening effects are underlined, generic names are in **bold,** and drug classes are in SMALL CAPS.

- Benzodiazepines or sedative-hypnotic drugs are withdrawn gradually before **buspirone** therapy is started. Observe for rebound symptoms which may occur at varying times.
- Involuntary movements may manifest in a small number of clients early in therapy. This includes dystonia, motor restlessness, and involuntary repetitive movement of facial and cervical muscle.
- Observe for swollen ankles, decreased urinary output, changes in voiding pattern along with symptoms of hepatic impairment (jaundice, itching, nausea, vomiting).

Client & Family Education

- **Buspirone** should be taken exactly as prescribed without dose omissions, skipping, increasing, or decreasing.
- Advice of prescriber should be sought prior to concomitant use of OTC medications.
- Therapeutic response may initiate in 7–10 d; optimal results are usually achieved in 3–4 weeks.
- Adverse and side effects occur early in therapy and subside without dosage changes.
- Cautious use of medication when client consumes alcohol.
- Rebound symptoms can occur at a low rate.

CHLORPROMAZINE (klor-proe′ma-zeen)

Trade names: Thorazine, Chlorpromanyl
Classifications: CNS AGENT; PSYCHOTHERAPEUTIC; PHENOTHIAZINE ANTIPSYCHOTIC; ANTIEMETIC
Pregnancy category: C

ACTIONS/PHARMACODYNAMICS Phenothiazine derivative with actions at all levels of CNS. Mechanism that produces strong antipsychotic effects is unclear, but thought to be related to blockade of postsynaptic dopamine receptors in the brain. Actions on hypothalamus and reticular formation produce strong sedation, hypotension, and depressed temperature regulation. Has strong alpha-adrenergic blocking action and weak anticholinergic effects. Directly depresses the heart; may increase coronary blood flow. Exerts quinidine-like antiarrhythmic action. Antiemetic effect by suppression of the chemoreceptor trigger zone (CTZ). Inhibitory effect on dopamine reuptake may be the basis for moderate extrapyramidal symptoms. Antipsychotic drugs are sometimes called neuroleptics because they tend to reduce initiative and interest in environment, decrease displays of emotion or affect, suppress spontaneous movements and complex behavior, and decrease psychotic symptoms. Spinal reflexes and unconditioned nociceptive-avoidance behaviors remain intact.

USES Symptom management of psychotic disorders, control manic phase of Bipolar Disorder, management of severe nausea and vomiting, control excessive preoperative anxiety and agitation, and treatment of severe behavioral problems in children.

ROUTE & DOSAGE
Psychotic Disorders, Agitation
Adult: 25–100 mg tid or qid; may need up to 1000 mg/d. **IM/IV** 25–50 mg up to 600 mg q4–6 h.

Child: >6 mo 0.55 mg/kg q4–6 h prn up to 500 mg/d. **PR** >6 mo 1.1 mg/kg q6–8 h. **IM/IV** >6 mo 0.55 mg/kg q6–8 h.
Nausea/Vomiting
Adult: 10–25 mg q4–6 prn. **PR** 50–100 mg q6–8 h. **IM/IV** 25–50 mg q3–4 h prn.

Child: >6 mo 0.55 mg/kg q4–6 h prn up to 500 mg/d. **PR** >6 mo 1.1 mg/kg q6–8 h. **IM/IV** >6 mo 0.55 mg/kg q6–8 h.

PHARMACOKINETICS
Absorption: rapid absorption with considerable first pass metabolism in liver; rapid absorption after IM.

Onset: 30–60 min.

Peak: 2–4 h PO, 15–20 min IM.

Duration: 4–6 h.

Distribution: widely distributed; accumulates in brain; crosses placenta.

Metabolism: metabolized in liver.

Elimination: half-life biphasic 2 and 30 h excreted in urine as metabolites, excreted in breast milk.

CONTRAINDICATIONS & PRECAUTIONS
Contradicted in: hypersensitivity to phenothiazine derivatives; withdrawal states from alcohol; comatose states, brain damage, bone marrow depression, Reye's Syndrome; children <6 mo. Safe use during pregnancy (category C), and in nursing mothers not established.

Cautious use in: agitated states accompanied by depression, seizure disorders, respiratory impairment due to infection or

COPD; glaucoma, diabetes, hypertensive disease, peptic ulcer, prostatic hypertrophy; thyroid, hepatic and cardiovascular disorders; clients exposed to extreme heat or organophosphate insecticides; previously detected breast cancer.

ADVERSE/SIDE EFFECTS Usually dose related. **CNS:** *sedation, drowsiness,* dizziness, restlessness, *neuroleptic malignant syndrome*; tardive dyskinesia, tumor, syncope, headache weakness, insomnia, reduced REM sleep, bizarre dreams, cerebral edema, seizures, *hypothermia,* inability to sweat, depressed cough reflex, *extrapyramidal symptoms,* EEG changes. **CV**: orthostatic hypotension, palpitation, tachycardia, ECG changes (usually reversible); prolonged QT and PR intervals blunting of T waves, ST depression. **Eye:** blurred vision, lenticular opacities, mydriasis, photophobia. **GI:** dry mouth, constipation, *adynamic ileus,* cholestatic jaundice, aggravation of peptic ulcer, dyspepsia, increased appetite. **GU:** anovulation, infertility, pseudopregnancy, menstrual irregularity, gynecomastia, galactorrhea, priapism, inhibition of ejaculation, reduced libido, urinary retention and frequency. **Hemotologic:** *agranulocytosis*, thrombocytopenia, purpura, *pancytopenia* (rare). **Respiratory:** laryngospasm. **Skin/hypersensitivity:** fixed-drug eruption, urticaria, reduced perspiration, contact dermatitis, exfoliative dermatitis, photosensitivity, eczema, anaphylactoid reactions, hypersensitivity vasculitis, hirsutism (long-term therapy). **Other:** weight gain, hypoglycemia, hyperglycemia, glycosuria (high doses), enlargement of parotid glands, idiopathic edema, muscle necrosis (following IM), SLE-like syndrome, *sudden unexplained death*.

DIAGNOSTIC TEST INTERFERENCE Chlorpromazine (phenothiazines) may increase cephalin flocculation, and possibly other *liver function tests;* also may increase **PBI**. False-positive result may occur for **amylase, 5-hydroxyindole acetic acid, porphobilinogens, urobilinogen** (Ehrlich's reagent) and **urine bilirubin** (Bili-Labstix). False-positive or false-negative **pregnancy test** results possibly caused by a metabolite of phenothiazines, which discolors urine depending on test used.

DRUG INTERACTIONS Alcohol, CNS DEPRESSANTS increase CNS depression; ANTACIDS ANTIDIARRHEALS decrease absorption—space administration 2h before or after administration of **chlorpromazine; phenobarbital** increases metabolism of phenothiazine; GENERAL ANESTHETICS increase excitation and hypotension; antagonizes antihypertensive action of **guanethidine; phenylpropanolamine** poses possibility of sudden death; TRICYCLIC ANTI-

DEPRESSANTS intensify hypotensive and anticholinergic effects; ANTICONVULSANTS decrease seizure threshold—may need to increase anticonvulsant dose.

Incompatibilities: Check for numerous solution and additive incompatible compounds.

NURSING IMPLICATIONS

Administration

- Concentrate to be mixed with liquid or semi-solid food immediately prior to administration.
- Administer IM preparation slowly and deeply into muscle. Avoid SC injection, as it may cause tissue irritation and nodule formation.

Assessment & Intervention

- Establish baseline pulse, respiratory capacity, and standing and recumbent BP prior to initiating therapy.
- Hypotensive reactions, dizziness, and sedation are common during early phases of treatment.
- Be alert for signs of neuroleptic malignant syndrome (NMS).
- Cigarette smoking increases the metabolism of phenothiazines, resulting in shorter half-lives and more rapid clearance of drug.
- Chlorpromazine can suppress cough reflex.
- Minimize drug-induced hypotension through support hose, elevation of legs while sitting.
- Track urine and blood glucose regularly with prediabetics and diabetics on long-term or high dose therapy for reduced glucose tolerance and loss of diabetes control.
- Monitor for early signs of agranulocytosis.

Client & Family Education

- Gastric irritation is reduced when medication taken with food or a full glass of water.
- Improvement may be seen as late as 7–8 weeks after starting medication regimen.
- May cause pink to red-brown discoloration of the urine.
- Monitor for phototoxic reactions such as sunburn and photosensitivity.
- Meticulous oral hygiene reduces risk of oral candidiasis.
- Educate regarding extrapyramidal side effects, reporting, treatment, and likelihood of occurrence.

Common side effects are shown in *italic,* life-threatening effects are underlined, generic names are in **bold,** and drug classes are in SMALL CAPS.

- Abrupt withdrawal or discontinuation of medication can cause extrapyramidal symptoms and severe GI disturbances.

FLUOXETINE (flu'-ox-e-tine)
Trade name: Prozac
Prototype for classifications: CNS AGENT; PSYCHOTHERAPEUTIC; SEROTONIN REUPTAKE INHIBITOR
Pregnancy category: B

ACTIONS/PHARMACODYNAMICS Oral antidepressant chemically unrelated to tricyclic, tetracyclic, or other available antidepressants. Antidepressant effect is presumed to be linked to its inhibition of CNS presynaptic neuronal uptake of serotonin.

USES Depression, obsessive–compulsive disorders, bulimia nervosa. Off label use: obesity.

ROUTE & DOSAGE
Depression
Adult: 20 mg/d in am; may increase to max of 80 mg/d.
Geriatric: may need to start with 10 mg/d.

PHARMACOKINETICS
Absorption: 60–80% absorbed from GI tract.
Onset: 1–3 wk.
Peak: 4–8 h.
Distribution: widely distributed, including CNS.
Metabolism: metabolized in liver to active metabolite, norfluoxetine.
Elimination: half-life fluoxetine 2–3 d, norfluoxetine 7–9 d; > 80% excreted in urine; 12% in feces.

CONTRAINDICATIONS & PRECAUTIONS
Contraindicated in: hypersensitivity to fluoxetine.
Cautious use in: hepatic and renal impairment, anorexia, hyponatremia, diabetes, and clients with history of suicidal ideations. Elderly may require dose adjustments. Safety in pregnancy (category B), lactation, and in children not established.

ADVERSE/SIDE EFFECTS **CNS:** *headache, nervousness, anxiety, insomnia,* drowsiness, fatigue, tremor, dizziness. **CV:** palpitations, hot flushes, chest pain. **GI:** *nausea, diarrhea,* anorexia, dyspepsia,

---

Common side effects are shown in *italic,* life-threatening effects are <u>underlined,</u> generic names are in **bold,** and drug classes are in SMALL CAPS.

increased appetite, dry mouth. **Skin:** rash, pruritus, sweating, hypersensitivity reactions. **Other:** blurred vision, myalgias, arthralgias, flu-like syndrome, hyponatremia, sexual dysfunction, menstrual irregularities.

DRUG INTERACTIONS Concurrent use of **tryptophan** may cause agitation, restlessness, and GI distress; MAO INHIBITORS, **selegiline** may increase risk of severe hypertensive reaction and death; increases half-life of **diazepam;** may increase toxicity of TRICYCLIC ANTIDEPRESSANTS.

NURSING IMPLICATIONS
Administration
- Administer single dose in AM. Any additional doses should be administered at noon.
- Assure that suicidal or potentially suicidal clients have small quantities of prescription medications.

Assessment & Intervention
- Use with caution in elderly client and client with impaired renal or hepatic function (may need lower dose).
- Use with caution in anorexic client, since weight loss is a possible side effect.
- Monitor for signs and symptoms of anaphylactoid or allergic reaction.
- Monitor for signs of improved affect. Requires approximately 2–3 wk for therapeutic effects to be felt.
- Weigh weekly to monitor weight loss, particularly in the elderly or nutritionally compromised client. Report significant weight loss to health care provider.
- Observe for and promptly report rash or urticaria and signs and symptoms of fever, leukocytosis, arthralgias, carpal tunnel syndrome, edema, respiratory distress, and proteinuria. Drug may have to be discontinued or adjunctive therapy instituted with steroids or antihistamines.
- Observe for dizziness and drowsiness and employ safety measures (ambulate with assistance, side rails, etc.) as indicated.
- Observe for and report increased anxiety, nervousness, or insomnia; modification of drug dose may be needed.
- Observe for seizures in clients with a history of seizures. Use appropriate safety precautions.

Common side effects are shown in *italic,* life-threatening effects are underlined, generic names are in **bold,** and drug classes are in SMALL CAPS.

- Closely supervise clients who are high suicide risks, especially during initial therapy.
- Carefully monitor clients with hepatic or renal impairment for signs of toxicity (e.g., agitation, restlessness, nausea, vomiting, seizures).
- Monitor serum sodium level for development of hyponatremia, especially in clients who are taking diuretics or are otherwise hypovolemic.
- Monitor diabetics for loss of control; hypoglycemia has occurred during initiation of therapy, and hyperglycemia during drug withdrawal.

Client & Family Education

- Instruct client to take medication in AM for single dose or AM and noon for divided doses, to prevent insomnia.
- Instruct client that therapeutic effects may take from several days to 5 wk to develop fully.
- Advise client to notify prescriber of intent to become pregnant or if breast feeding.
- Instruct client that a rash could be one sign of a serious group of adverse effects and to notify prescriber if noted.
- Caution clients, particularly the elderly, to exercise safety precautions and to avoid hazardous tasks if dizziness noted.
- Advise diabetics of possible loss of diabetic control and need for careful monitoring.
- Advise those with history of seizures of possible increase in seizure activity.

LITHIUM (li-'thee-um)
Trade names: Carbolith, Eskalith, Lithobid, Lithonate
Classifications: CNS AGENT; PSYCHOTHERAPEUTIC; ANTIMANIC
Pregnancy category: D

ACTIONS/PHARMACODYNAMICS Affects cell membranes, body water, and neurotransmitters. At the synapse, it accelerates catecholamine destruction, inhibits the release of neurotransmitters, and decreases sensitivity of postsynaptic receptors. Thus, neurotransmitter overactivity assumed to occur in mania is corrected. Has antidepressant and antimanic effects.

USES Control and prophylaxis of acute mania and the acute manic phase of mixed bipolar disorder.

Common side effects are shown in *italic*, life-threatening effects are <u>underlined</u>, generic names are in **bold**, and drug classes are in SMALL CAPS.

ROUTE & DOSAGE
Mania
Adult: initial: 600 mg t.i.d. or 900 sustained release b.i.d. or 30 ml (48 mEq) of solution t.i.d.
Maintenance: 300 mg t.i.d. or q.i.d. or 15–20 ml (24–32 mEq) solution in 2–4 divided doses (max 2.4 g/d).
Child: 15–60 mg/kg/d in divided doses.

PHARMACOKINETICS
Absorption: readily absorbed from GI tract.
Peak: 0.5–3h.
lithium carbonate.
Distribution: crosses blood-brain barrier and placenta; distributed into breast milk.
Metabolism: not metabolized.
Elimination: half-life 20–27 h; 95% excreted in urine, 1% in feces, 4–5% in sweat.

CONTRAINDICATIONS & PRECAUTIONS
Contraindicated in: significant cardiovascular or renal disease, brain damage, severe debilitation, dehydration or sodium depletion; people on low salt diet or receiving diuretics; pregnancy, especially first trimester (category D), nursing mothers, children <12 y.
Cautious use in: elderly people, thyroid disease, epilepsy; concomitant use with **haloperidol** and other antipsychotics; Parkinsonism; diabetes mellitus; severe infections; urinary retention.

ADVERSE/SIDE EFFECTS
CNS: dizziness, *headache, lethargy,* drowsiness, *fatigue,* slurred speech, psychomotor retardation, giddiness, incontinence, restlessness, seizures, confusion, blackout spells, disorientation, *recent memory loss,* stupor, coma, EEG changes. **CV:** arrhythmias, hypotension, vasculitis, *peripheral circulatory collapse*, ECG changes. **EENT:** impaired vision, transient scotomas, tinnitus. **Endocrine:** diffuse thyroid enlargement, hypothyroidism, *nephrogenic diabetes insipidus,* transient hyperglycemia, glycosuria, hyponatremia. **GI:** *nausea, vomiting, anorexia, abdominal pain, diarrhea, dry mouth,* metallic taste. **Neuromuscular:** *fine hand tremors,* coarse tremors, choreoathetetic movements, fasciculations, clonic movements, incoordination including ataxia, *muscle weakness,* hyperreflexia, encephalopathic syndrome (weakness, lethargy, fever, tremors, confusion, extrapyramidal symptoms). **Skin:** pruritus, maculopapular rash,

---

Common side effects are shown in *italic*, life-threatening effects are underlined, generic names are in **bold**, and drug classes are in SMALL CAPS.

hyperkeratosis, chronic folliculitis, transient acneiform papules (face, neck, intertriginous areas), anesthesia of skin, cutaneous ulcers, drying and thinning of the hair, allergic vasculitis. **Other:** *reversible leukocytosis* (14,000–18,000/mm^3), albuminuria, oliguria, urinary incontinence, polyuria, polydipsia, increased uric acid excretion, edema, weight gain or loss, exacerbation of psoriasis, flu-like symptoms.

DRUG INTERACTIONS Carbamazepine, haloperidol, PHENOTHIAZINES increase risk of neurotoxicity, extrapyramidal effects and tardive dyskinesia; DIURETICS, NSAIDS, **methyldopa, probenecid,** TETRACYCLINES decrease renal clearance of lithium, increasing pharmacologic and toxic effects; THEOPHYLLINES, **urea, sodium bicarbonate, sodium or potassium citrate** increase renal clearance of lithium, decreasing its pharmacologic effects.

NURSING IMPLICATIONS

Administration

• Administer with meals to decrease GI symptoms.

Assessment & Intervention

• Therapeutic response seen in 1–2 weeks. Keep prescriber informed of signs of progress: changed facial affect, improved posture, assumption of self-care, improved ability to concentrate, improved sleep pattern.
• Monitor **lithium** level via blood sample taken 8–12 h after last dose. Note that effective and toxic range indicated by lithium level varies by race/culture/age.
• Note signs of **lithium** intoxication: vomiting, diarrhea, lack of coordination, drowsiness, muscular weakness, slurred speech. Hold one dose; notify prescriber; do not stop drug abruptly.
• Signs of toxic levels: ataxia, blurred vision, giddiness, tinnitus, muscle twitching or coarse tremors, and a large output of dilute urine.
• Neonates born of mothers who took **lithium** during pregnancy may have high serum lithium levels manifested by flaccidity, poor reflexes, cardiac dysrhythmia, and chronic twitching.

Client & Family Education

• Instruct to be alert to increased output of dilute urine and persistent thirst.
• Because dehydration is possible, contact prescriber if diarrhea or fever develops.

Common side effects are shown in *italic,* life-threatening effects are <u>underlined</u>, generic names are in **bold,** and drug classes are in SMALL CAPS.

- Urge drinking 2–3 L/d of fluids during stabilization on **lithium,**
  1–1.5 L/d thereafter.
- Normal dietary salt intake can be inadvertently compromised
  by self-prescribing a low-salt diet; self-dosing with Rolaids,
  soda-mints, or other sodium antacid; and high sodium foods.
- Review need for contraception, risks to fetus, close monitoring
  of **lithium** level during pregnancy, high renal clearance of
  lithium during pregnancy and lower rate clearance immediately following delivery with associated dosage adjustments to
  prevent toxicity.
- Warn against switching brands of **lithium.** Different fillers may
  require dosage adjustments.

NEFAZADONE (nef-a-zo′done)
Trade name: Serzone
Classifications: CNS AGENT; PSYCHOTHERAPEUTIC; SEROTONIN REUP-
TAKE INHIBITOR; ANTIDEPRESSANT
Pregnancy category: C

ACTIONS/PHARMACODYNAMICS Nefazodone is an antidepressant with a dual mechanism of action. It inhibits neuronal serotonin (5-HT) reuptake and also possesses 5-HT2 antagonist properties. It is unrelated to tricyclic, MAO, or other antidepressants.
Nefazodone has minimal cardiovascular effects, fewer anticholer-
genic effects, less sedation, and less sexual dysfunction than
other antidepressants.

USE Treatment of depression.

ROUTE & DOSAGE
Depression
Adult: 50–100 mg b.i.d.; may need to increase up to 300–600
mg/d in 2–3 divided doses.
Elderly: start elderly clients with 50 mg b.i.d.

PHARMACOKINETICS
Onset: 1 wk.
Peak: 3–5 wk.
Metabolism: metabolized in liver to at least two active metabo-
lites.
Elimination: half-life **nefazodone** 3.5 h, metabolites 2–33 h.

Common side effects are shown in *italic,* life-threatening effects are <u>underlined</u>,
generic names are in **bold,** and drug classes are in SMALL CAPS.

CONTRAINDICATIONS & PRECAUTIONS
Contraindicated in: hypersensitivity to nefazodone or alcohol.
Cautious use in: elderly, women, history of seizure disorders, renal and hepatic impairment, pregnancy (category C), nursing mothers. Safety and efficacy in children <18 y have not been established.

ADVERSE/SIDE EFFECTS **CNS:** *headache, dizziness, drowsiness,* asthenia, tremor, insomnia, agitation, anxiety. **GI:** dry mouth, constipation, nausea.

DRUG INTERACTIONS May increase plasma levels of some BENZODIAZEPINES, including **alprazolam** and **triazolam.** May decrease plasma levels and effects of **propranolol.** May increase levels and toxicity of **carbamazepine, digoxin.**

NURSING IMPLICATIONS
Administration
- Dosage adjustment may be warranted with elderly clients.
- Store at room temperature, 15–30C (59–86F).

Assessment & Intervention
- Monitor clients with a history of seizures for increased activity.
- Assess safety, as dizziness and drowsiness are common adverse effects.
- Periodically monitor HR, BP, hepatic function tests, and CBC during long-term therapy.

Client & Family Education
- Advise that significant improvement in mood may not occur for several weeks following initiation of therapy.
- Caution about performing hazardous activities until response to the drug is known.
- Advise client to report changes in visual acuity.

OLANZAPINE (o-lan'za-peen)
Trade name: Zyprexa
Classifications: CNS AGENT, PSYCHOTHERAPEUTIC, NEUROLEPTIC AGENT, SEROTONIN REUPTAKE INHIBITOR, DOPAMINE REUPTAKE INHIBITOR
Pregnancy category: C

Common side effects are shown in *italic,* life-threatening effects are <u>underlined,</u> generic names are in **bold,** and drug classes are in SMALL CAPS.

ACTIONS/PHARMACODYNAMICS Antipsychotic activity thought to be due to antagonism for both serotonin $5HT_{2A/2C}$ and dopamine D_{1-4} receptors. Is thought to inhibit the CNS presynaptic neuronal reuptake of serotonin and dopamine. Antagonism of alpha-adrenergic receptors results in the side effect of orthostatic hypotension. Also has anticholinergic properties.

USES Management of psychotic disorders, short-term treatment of acute manic episodes from bipolar I disorder.

ROUTE & DOSAGE
Psychotic Disorders
Adult: start with 5–10 mg qd, may increase by 2.5–5 mg qwk until desired response (usually 10–15 mg/d), max 20 mg/d.
Geriatric: start with 5 mg qd.
Manic Episode
Adults: initially 10–15 mg daily. Adjust dosage as needed in increments of 5 mg daily at intervals of 24 h or more. Max 20 mg/d. Duration of treatment 3–4 weeks.

PHARMACOKINETICS
Absorption: rapidly absorbed from GI tract; 60% reaches systemic circulation.
Peak: 6 h.
Distribution: 93% protein bound, secreted into breast milk of animals (human secretion unknown).
Metabolism: metabolized in liver, primarily by cytochrome $P_{450}1A2$ (CYP1A2).
Elimination: half-life 21–54 h; approximately 57% excreted in urine, 30% in feces.

CONTRAINDICATIONS & PRECAUTIONS
Contraindicated in: hypersensitivity to **olanzapine,** lactation.
Cautious use in: known cardiovascular disease, conditions that predispose to hypotension, history of breast cancer, hepatic or renal impairment, predisposition to aspiration pneumonia, history of or high risk of suicide, pregnancy (category C). Safety and efficacy in children <18 y not established.

ADVERSE/SIDE EFFECTS Body as whole: *weight gain,* fever, back and chest pain, peripheral and lower extremity edema, joint pain, twitching, premenstrual syndrome. Neuroleptic malignant syndrome **CNS:** *somnolence, dizziness, headache, agitation, insomnia, nervousness, hostility,* anxiety cognitive impairment, per-

Common side effects are shown in *italic,* life-threatening effects are <u>underlined,</u> generic names are in **bold,** and drug classes are in SMALL CAPS.

sonality disorder, akathisia, hypertonia, tremor, amnesia, euphoria, stuttering, extrapyramidal symptoms, tardive dyskinesia. **CV:** postural hypotension, hypotension, tachycardia. **Eye:** amblyopia, blepharitis. **GI:** abdominal pain, constipation, dry mouth, increased appetite, increased salivation, nausea, vomiting, elevated liver function tests. **GU:** premenstrual syndrome, hematuria, urinary incontinence, metrorrhagia. **Respiratory:** rhinitis, cough, pharyngitis, dyspnea. **Skin:** rash.

DRUG INTERACTIONS May enhance hypotensive effects of ANTI-HYPERTENSIVES. May enhance effects of other CNS active drugs; **alcohol, carbamazepine, omeprazole, rifampin** may increase metabolism and clearance of olanzapine. **Fluvoxamine** may inhibit metabolism and clearance of **olanzapine.**

NURSING IMPLICATIONS

Assessment & Intervention

- Withhold drug and immediately report signs of neuroleptic malignant syndrome (NMS).
- Assess and report signs of tardive dyskinesia. Periodically monitor ALT/SGPT, especially in those with hepatic dysfunction or being treated with other potentially hepatotoxic drugs.
- Monitor for seizures.
- Actively involve client in weight management philosophy upon initiation of medication to minimize impact of weight gain side effect.

Client & Family Education

- Warn of risk for orthostatic hypotension and cognitive impairment.
- Educate on common side effects and drug interactions.
- Instruct to avoid alcohol and take no additional medications (especially OTC) prior to discussion with prescriber.
- Mothers should not breastfeed while on **olanzapine.**
- Advise against overheating and conditions leading to dehydration.

RISPERIDONE (ris-per'-i-done)
Trade name: Risperdal
Classifications: CNS AGENT; ANTIPSYCHOTIC; NEUROLEPTIC AGENT
Pregnancy category: C

Common side effects are shown in *italic,* life-threatening effects are <u>underlined</u>, generic names are in **bold,** and drug classes are in SMALL CAPS.

ACTIONS/PHARMACODYNAMICS Mechanism is not defined. Interferes with binding of dopamine to D2-interlimbic region of the brain, serotonin (5-HT2) receptors, and alpha-adrenergic receptors in the occipital cortex. It has low to moderate affinity to the other serotonin (5-HT) receptors and no affinity to nondopaminergic sites (e.g., cholinergic, muscarinic, or beta-adrenergic receptors).

USES Reduction or elimination of psychotic symptoms in schizophrenia and related psychoses. Seems to improve negative symptoms such as apathy, blunted affect, and emotional withdrawal. Off label use: dementia, mania, adjunctive treatment of behavioral disturbances in clients with mental retardation.

ROUTE & DOSAGE
Psychosis
Adult: 1–6 mg b.i.d. Begin with 1 mg b.i.d., increase by 1 mg b.i.d. daily to an initial target dose of 3 mg b.i.d.
Elderly, debilitated, and clients with renal insufficiency: Start with 0.5 mg b.i.d. and increase by 0.5 mg b.i.d. daily to an initial target of 1.5 mg b.i.d. (max 6 mg/d).

PHARMACOKINETICS
Absorption: rapidly absorbed; not affected by food.
Onset: therapeutic effect 1–2 wk.
Peak: 1–2 h.
Distribution: 0.7 L/kg; in animal studies, risperidone has been found in breast milk.
Metabolism: metabolized primarily in liver by cytochrome P450 with an active metabolite, 9-hydroxyrisperidone.
Elimination: half-life 20h for fast metabolizers, 30h for slow metabolizers; 70% excreted in urine; 15% in feces.

CONTRAINDICATIONS & PRECAUTIONS
Contraindicated in: hypersensitivity to **risperidone,** lactation.
Cautious use in: arrhythmias, hypotension, history of seizures, breast cancer, blood dyscrasia, cardiac disorders, renal or hepatic impairment, pregnancy (category C). Safety and efficacy in children not established.

ADVERSE/SIDE EFFECTS CNS: *sedation, drowsiness*, headache, transient blurred vision, fatigue, insomnia, disinhibition, agitation,

Common side effects are shown in *italic,* life-threatening effects are <u>underlined</u>, generic names are in **bold,** and drug classes are in SMALL CAPS.

dizziness, catatonia. **GI:** dry mouth, constipation. **Other:** urinary retention, tachycardia, elevated liver function tests (AST, ALT), sweating, weakness.

DIAGNOSTIC TEST INTERFERENCE Liver function tests **(AST, ALT)** are elevated.

DRUG INTERACTIONS Risperidone may enhance the effects of certain ANTIHYPERTENSIVE AGENTS. May antagonize the effects of **levodopa** and dopamine agonists. **Carbamazepine** may decrease risperidone levels. **Clozapine** may increase **risperidone** levels.

NURSING IMPLICATIONS

Administration

- When dosage adjustments are made, increases/decreases should not exceed 1 mg b.i.d. in normal populations and 0.5 mg b.i.d. in the elderly or debilitated.
- When the target doses of 3 mg b.i.d. in normal populations and 1.5 mg b.i.d. in the elderly or debilitated are reached, further increases should be made at 1-wk or longer intervals.
- Store at room temperature, 15–30C (59–86F).

Assessment & Intervention

- Clients should be reassessed periodically and maintained on the lowest effective drug dose.
- Closely monitor cardiovascular status; assess for orthostatic hypotension, especially during initial dosage titration.
- Assess degree of cognitive and motor impairment, and assess for environmental hazards.
- Periodically monitor serum electrolytes, liver function tests, and complete blood counts.

Client & Family Education

- Advise to exercise caution with hazardous activities until the reaction to the drug is known.
- Advise of adverse drug effects and instruct to report those that are bothersome.
- Discuss the risk of orthostatic hypotension with the client.
- Advise to wear sunscreen and protective clothing to avoid photosensitivity.
- Advise female clients to notify prescriber if they intend to become or have become pregnant.

Common side effects are shown in *italic,* life-threatening effects are <u>underlined,</u> generic names are in **bold,** and drug classes are in SMALL CAPS.

TRAZODONE (tray'zoe-done)
Trade names: Desyrel, Desyrel Dividose
Classifications: CNS AGENT; PSYCHOTHERAPEUTIC; ANTIDEPRESSANT
Pregnancy category: C

ACTIONS/PHARMACODYNAMICS Centrally acting triazolepyri-
dine derivative antidepressant chemically and structurally unrelated to tricyclic, tetracyclic, or other antidepressants. Potentiates
serotonin effects by selectively blocking its reuptake at presynaptic
membranes in CNS. Does not stimulate CNS and causes fewer
anticholinergic genitourinary and neurologic effects as compared
with other antidepressants. Produces varying degrees of sedation
in normal and mentally depressed client, increases total sleep
time, decreases number and duration of awakenings in depressed
client, and decreases REM sleep. Has anxiolytic effect in severely
depressed client.

USES Both inpatient and outpatient with major depression, with or
without prominent anxiety. Off label uses: adjunctive treatment of
alcohol dependence, anxiety neuroses, drug-induced dyskinesias.

ROUTE & DOSAGE
Depression
Adult: 150 mg/d in divided doses; may increase by 50 mg/d q3–4d
(max 400–600 mg/d).
Geriatric: 25–50 mg h.s., may increase q3–7d to usual range of
75–150 mg/d.
Child 6–18 y: 1.5–2 mg/kg/d in divided doses; increase q3–4d prn
(max 6 mg/kg/d).

PHARMACOKINETICS
Absorption: readily absorbed from GI tract.
Onset: 1–2 wk.
Peak: 1–2 h.
Distribution: distributed into breast milk.
Metabolism: metabolized in liver.
Elimination: half-life: 5–9 h; 75% excreted in urine, 25% in feces.

CONTRAINDICATIONS & PRECAUTIONS
Contraindicated in: initial recovery phase of MI, ventricular ec-
topy; electroshock therapy. Safe use in children <18 y not established; pregnancy (category C).

Common side effects are shown in *italic,* life-threatening effects are underlined,
generic names are in **bold,** and drug classes are in SMALL CAPS.

Cautious use in: client with suicidal ideation, cardiac arrhythmias or disease; nursing mother.

ADVERSE/SIDE EFFECTS Appear to be dose related. **CNS:** *drowsiness,* light-headedness, tiredness, dizziness, insomnia, headache, agitation, impaired memory and speech, disorientation. **CV:** *hypotension (including orthostatic hypotension),* hypertension, syncope, shortness of breath, chest pain, tachycardia, palpitations, bradycardia, PVCs, ventricular tachycardia (short episodes of 3–4 beats). **ENT:** nasal and sinus congestion, blurred vision, eye irritation, sweating or clamminess, tinnitus. **GI:** *dry mouth,* anorexia, constipation, abdominal distress, nausea, vomiting, dysgeusia, flatulence, diarrhea. **GU:** hematuria, increased frequency, delayed urine flow, early or absent menses, male priapism, ejaculation inhibition. **Hematologic:** anemia. **Musculoskeletal:** skeletal aches and pains, muscle twitches. Skin: skin eruptions, rash, pruritus, acne, photosensitivity. **Other:** weight gain or loss.

DRUG INTERACTIONS ANTIHYPERTENSIVE AGENTS may potentiate hypotensive effects; **alcohol** and other CNS DEPRESSANTS add to depressant effects; may increase **digoxin** or **phenytoin** levels; MAO INHIBITORS may precipitate hypertensive crisis.

NURSING IMPLICATIONS

Administration

- Taking drug with food increases amount of absorption by 20% and appears to decrease incidence of dizziness or light-headedness. Urge client to maintain the same schedule for food–drug intake throughout treatment period to prevent variations in serum concentration.
- Store in tightly closed, light-resistant container at 15–30C (59–86F).

Assessment & In tervention

- If client has preexisting cardiac disease, monitor pulse rate and regularity before administration of drug.
- When trazodone is given concurrently with an MAO inhibitor, therapy is initiated cautiously, and dose is adjusted according to clinical response. No interaction has been documented, but the potential for hypertensive crisis is recognized until ruled out.

Common side effects are shown in *italic,* life-threatening effects are <u>underlined,</u>
generic names are in **bold,** and drug classes are in SMALL CAPS.

- Adverse/side effects generally are mild and tend to decrease and disappear after the first few weeks of treatment.
- Observe client's level of activity. If it appears to be increasing toward sleeplessness and agitation with changes in reality orientation, report to prescriber. Manic episodes have been reported.
- Check client for symptoms of hypotension. If orthostatic hypotension is troublesome, suggest measures to reduce danger of falling and to help client to tolerate the effects. Discuss with prescriber; a reduction of dose or discontinuation of the drug may be prescribed.
- Ask male client if he is having inappropriate or prolonged penile erections. If he is, the drug should be discontinued and prescriber consulted.
- Overdose is characterized by an extension of common adverse/side effects: vomiting, lethargy, drowsiness, and exaggerated anticholinergic effects. Seizures or arrhythmias are unusual. Death rarely occurs except when other drugs are being taken concomitantly (such as alcohol, meprobamate).

Client & Family Education

- Therapeutic effects usually begin in 1 wk but may require 2–4 wk to reach maximum levels. Teach client importance of adhering to regimen and have family member reinforce this teaching with client in the home.
- Urge not to alter dose or intervals between doses.
- If drowsiness becomes a distressing side effect, client should consult prescriber. Dose regimen may be adjusted so that largest dose is at bedtime.
- Advise to limit or abstain from alcohol use. The depressant effects of CNS depressants and alcohol may be potentiated by this drug.
- Warn not to self-medicate with OTC drugs for colds, allergy, or insomnia treatment without advice of health care provider. Many of these drugs contain CNS depressants.
- Adherence to follow-up appointment is important to permit dose adjustment or discontinuation, as indicated.
- Alert dentist, surgeon, or emergency personnel that drug is being used. Trazodone is discontinued as long as possible prior to elective surgery.

Common side effects are shown in *italic,* life-threatening effects are <u>underlined</u>, generic names are in **bold,** and drug classes are in SMALL CAPS.

VALPROIC ACID (val-proe'ic) (divalproex sodium, sodium valproate)
Trade names: Depacon, Depakene, Depakote, Depakote ER, Depakote Sprinkle
Pregnancy category: D

ACTIONS/PHARMACODYNAMICS Anticonvulsant unrelated chemically to other drugs used to treat seizure disorders. Mechanism of action unknown; may be related to increased bioavailability of the inhibitory neurotransmitter GABA to brain neurons. Inhibits secondary phase of platelet aggregation.

USES Alone or with other anticonvulsants in management of absence (petit mal) and mixed seizures; mania; migraine headache prophylaxis. Off label uses: other types of seizures including psychomotor (temporal lobe), myoclonic, akinetic and tonic-clonic seizures, photosensitivity seizures.

ROUTE & DOSAGE
Management of Seizures, Mania
Adult/child: IV 15 mg/kg/d in divided doses when total daily dose > 250 mg; increase at 1 wk intervals by 5–10 mg/kg/d until seizures are controlled or side effects develop (max 60 mg/ kg/d).
Migraine Headache Prophylaxis
Adult: 250 mg b.i.d., may increase to max of 1000 mg/d; or Depakote ER 500 mg q.d. ×
1 week, may increase to 1000 mg q.d.
Mania
Adult: 250 mg t.i.d., may increase to max of 60 mg/kg/d.

PHARMACOKINETICS
Absorption: readily absorbed from GI tract.
Peak: 1–4 h **valproic acid;** 3–5 h **divalproex.**
Therapeutic range: 50–100 g/ml.
Distribution: crosses placenta; distributed into breast milk.
Metabolism: metabolized in liver.
Elimination: half-life 5–20 h; excreted primarily in urine; small amount excreted in feces and expired air.

CONTRAINDICATIONS & PRECAUTIONS
Contraindicated in: client with bleeding disorders or hepatic dysfunction or disease, pregnancy (category D), nursing mothers.

Common side effects are shown in *italic,* life-threatening effects are <u>underlined</u>, generic names are in **bold,** and drug classes are in SMALL CAPS.

Cautious use in: history of renal disease; adjunctive treatment with other anticonvulsants.

ADVERSE/SIDE EFFECTS

CNS: breakthrough seizures, *sedation, drowsiness,* dizziness, increased alertness, hallucinations, emotional upset, aggression. **GI:** *nausea, vomiting, indigestion (transient),* hypersalivation, anorexia with weight loss, increased appetite with weight gain, abdominal cramps, diarrhea, constipation, *hepatic failure,* pancreatitis (lt). **Hematologic:** *prolonged bleeding time*, leukopenia, lymphocytosis, thrombocytopenia, hypofibrinogenemia, bone marrow depression, anemia. **Other:** skin rash, transient hair loss, curliness or waviness of hair, irregular menses, secondary amenorrhea, photosensitivity; hyperammonemia (usually asymptomatic).**Overdosage:** deep coma, pulmonary edema, death.

DIAGNOSTIC TEST INTERFERENCE Valproic acid produces false-positive results for *urine ketones*, elevated *AST, ALT, LDH,* and *serum alkaline phosphatase, prolonged bleeding time*, altered *thyroid function* tests.

DRUG INTERACTIONS Alcohol and other CNS DEPRESSANTS potentiate depressant effects; other anticonvulsants, barbiturates increase levels and toxicity; **aspirin, dipyridamole, warfarin** increase risk of spontaneous bleed and decrease clotting; **clonazepam** may precipitate absence seizures; **salicylates, cimetidine** may increase **valproic acid** levels and toxicity. **Cholestyramine** may decrease absorption. Herb: **Ginko** may decrease anticonvulsant effectiveness.

NURSING IMPLICATIONS

Administration

- Tablets and capsules should not be chewed. Medication should be swallowed whole. Client should avoid using a carbonated drink as diluent for the syrup because it will release drug from delivery vehicle. Free drug painfully irritates oral and pharyngeal membranes.
- Serious GI side effects can lead to discontinuation of therapy with **valproic acid.** To reduce gastric irritation, administer drug with food. Enteric-coated tablet or syrup formulation is usually well tolerated.
- Abrupt discontinuation of therapy can lead to increased risk of seizures. Warn client not to stop or alter dosage regimen without consulting prescriber.

Assessment & Intervention

- Effective therapeutic serum levels of **valproic acid** are 50–100 µg/ml.
- Increased dosage increases frequency of adverse effects. Monitor client carefully when dose adjustments are being made and report promptly if side effects persist.
- Platelet counts and bleeding time determinations are recommended prior to initiating treatment and at periodic intervals. Liver function tests, including serum ammonia, should be performed initially and at least q2mo, especially during the first 6 mo of therapy.

Client & Family Education

- Inform the diabetic client that this drug may cause a false-positive test for urine ketones. Should that occur, notify health care provider; a differential diagnostic blood test may be indicated.
- If spontaneous bleeding or bruising (petechiae, ecchymotic areas, otorrhagia, epistaxis, melena) occurs, notify health care provider promptly.
- Instruct to withhold dose and report to the prescriber if the following symptoms appear: visual disturbances, rash, jaundice, light-colored stools, protracted vomiting, diarrhea. Fatal hepatic failure has occurred in clients receiving this drug.
- Warn to avoid alcohol and self-medication with other depressants during therapy. The use of all OTC drugs should be approved by the prescriber. Particularly unsafe are combination drugs containing aspirin, sedatives, and medications for hay fever or other allergies.
- Advise not to drive a car or engage in other activities requiring mental alertness and physical coordination until reaction to drug is known.
- Before any kind of surgery (including dental surgery), the client should inform the doctor or dentist about taking **valproic acid.**
- Advise to carry medical identification card or jewelry bearing information about medication in use and the epilepsy diagnosis.

IV

CLINICAL
APPLICATIONS

AGGRESSIVE CLIENT: PHYSICAL/VERBAL

There is increasing recognition in society and in nursing that anger and violence are significant health problems. Violence is also an ever-increasing problem in health care environments. According to the Occupational Safety and Health Administration (OSHA, 2000), the highest number of nonfatal assaults in the workplace were on nursing staff in health care institutions. Accurate assessment and early intervention are of primary importance when dealing with verbally or physically aggressive clients.

Assessment Cues

- Take a comprehensive violence history on admission to identify patterns or trends in angry and violent behaviors and the conditions under which an individual is likely to respond with anger or violence
- Ask open and direct questions, as if you were questioning a suicidal individual (How often have you felt angry? What do you do when you are angry? How much have you thought about violence? What have you done about it?)
- Review the client's history and past records—do not rely solely on client responses
- Assess for the presence of substance abuse or medical problems such as temporal lobe epilepsy or brain tumor, since there is increased potential for aggressive behavior
- Observe the client for indicators of escalating anger or aggressiveness:

  Verbal
  - Threats of harm
  - Loud, demanding voice tone
  - Abrupt silence
  - Sarcastic remarks
  - Pressured speech
  - Illogical responses
  - Yelling, screaming
  - Statements of fear and/or
  - Suspicion

Behavioral
- Clenched jaws
- Frowning, glaring
- Intense staring
- Flushing of face and neck
- Smirking grin
- Dilated pupils
- Pacing
- Pounding fists
- Heightened vigilance
- Note the client's ability to solve problems and cope with stressors

Interventions

- Protect the client and others from harm. *The primary goal for all health care providers in every setting is maintenance of safety.*
- Set limits on inappropriate behavior by providing consistent expectations and guidelines for self-control. *Remember to use limit setting as a therapeutic intervention, not a punitive tool. Limit setting is a temporary process to protect the client and others.*
- Accept the client while rejecting the angry/violent behavior. *Protects self-esteem and reinforces behavioral limits.*
- Provide treatment in the least restrictive environment, while maintaining safety. *Balancing the need for safety maintenance with the need for assuring individual freedom of the violent client is ethically and legally responsible behavior and establishes a treatment environment that is client-focused and non-coercive.*
- Employ active listening. *Listening for the expression of unmet needs (such as needs for control and dependency), and for expression of the ability to regain/maintain control is important for early intervention.*
- Establish a therapeutic nurse–client relationship that demonstrates compassion and caring. *Establishing rapport helps reduce suspiciousness by building trust. When clients feel they are in a supportive relationship, there is less need to "prove" their superiority.*

- Make frequent, short, individualized contacts with the client. *Allows the client to temporarily withdraw from interpersonal demands, is reassuring, and may de-escalate a situation.*

- Be aware of, and try to decrease, dehumanizing and depersonalizing elements of the milieu. *Overcrowding, lack of privacy, and inflexibility of regulations regarding activities and programming contribute to a client's agitation, anger, fear, or feeling of being trapped.*

- Provide psychoeducation—anger management skills, social skills training, problem solving, communication skills training, assertiveness training, relaxation skills. *Psychoeducation empowers the client by providing tools for increasing self-responsibility and self-control.*

- Recognize that most angry or violent episodes involve an escalation of behavior and use the following de-escalation techniques before clients become out of control: diversion, exercise, change of surroundings, release from schedule or "demands," relaxation, music, quiet periods, being read to or talked to by staff, a quiet walk, citing phrases or counting, thought stopping (a cognitive–behavioral technique in which the client examines angry thoughts and feelings that drive action). *These de-escalation strategies are alternatives to the use of restrictive measures of control (such as seclusion and restraint) and help to avert a crisis.*

- Use clear, calm statements, and a confident physical stance. *It is important to convey control while avoiding a confrontational, aggressive, or threatening manner that can actually precipitate violence and make you a target.*

- Avoid touching clients when they are upset and posing an immediate danger. *Communicates respect for the client and maintains a comfortable distance, thereby reducing the client's sense of threat.*

- Reward desirable, nonviolent behaviors. *Focuses on the client's strength, maintains the client's self-esteem, and promotes continued demonstration of expected behavior(s).*

- When verbal interventions are insufficient to contain the situation, or when an assault occurs with warning, other interventions—such as medications, behavioral techniques, and seclusion and restraint—can be used with or instead of verbal strategies. Document efforts to intervene using verbal strategies, before intervening physically. *All interventions must be considered within the context of the principle of least restrictiveness.*

- Administer pharmacologic interventions—such as fluoxetine, paroxetine, haloperidol, thiothixene, fluphenazine, clozapine, risperidone, valproic acid. *These pharmacologic agents may reduce agitation and aggression. Remember that medications alone are not the answer to violence.*

- Implement behavioral strategies such as encouraging the client to seek quiet refuge at the back of the unit or in a private room or quiet room or other quiet, less active, nonstimulating environment. *Reduces disruptive stimulation and provides the client with a contained, well defined space for reassurance and protection; avoids the more restrictive procedures of seclusion and restraint.*

- Use seclusion and restraint applied by trained personnel, according to agency procedures, only upon the written order of a physician or other licensed practitioner, and only in the case of behavioral emergency. *The risk of injury to clients and staff is increased when physical restraints are applied. Asphyxiation and cardiac arrest have been associated with the use of psychiatric restraints.*

- Once a client is placed in seclusion or restraint, observe the client's behavior every 15 minutes. Describe and document the

---

Communicating with the Physically/ Verbally Aggressive Client

Client: Red in face, shaking fist at another client, yelling, and beginning to lift a chair. "Let me at him. Just let me at him. I'll show him what for."

Nurse: "Connie, walk with me now to the quiet room." *Rationale: Provides behavioral controls—the client uses energy walking to a quieter, less stimulating environment, and is removed from the precipitating situation, deflecting attention away from the client who has become the target for the violent behavior. This strategy assists in de-escalation.*	**Nurse:** Approaches client from the side while appearing confident. "Put the chair down, Connie. Now count to 20. We will help you to control yourself." *Rationale: Not standing face to face with a potentially violent person decreases the violent person's tendency to project and externalize the assault. Counting provides a diversion. Providing external controls promotes a sense of safety.*

client's behavior, routine activities, meals, circulation checks, and toileting. *Ensures the client's safety and provides data for the basis for the decision to release.*

- Teach family members, friends, and significant others the indicators for impending violence and specific techniques for defusing anger and violence. *Assists angry and aggressive clients to function in the community and provides family with a way to convey external controls.*

AGGRESSIVE CLIENT: SEXUAL

Sexual acting out is psychiatric jargon for overt sexual behavior on the part of either male or female clients.

Assessment Cues

- Making flirtatious comments
- Assess for sexual acting out behaviors
- Attempting to touch or hold a nurse
- Boasting about sexual experiences
- Deliberately exposing one's genitals
- Assess for threats to image of self as an active, sexual being
- Assess for regression—may be psychiatric in origin, or relate to hospitalization and the client role that encourages regressive behavior, regardless of type of hospital or facility
- Assess for emotional deprivation
- Assess for touch deprivation
- Assess for self-esteem disturbance
- Assess staff responses:
  1. Shunning the client
  2. Chastising the client verbally
  3. Criticizing the client to others
  4. Ignoring or pretending not to notice the behavior
  5. Considering the behavior as expected of a hospitalized person
  6. Considering the behavior inappropriate for some, and not for others (e.g., a young, attractive male who flirts may be acceptable while a paunchy, middle-aged man may be labeled "a dirty old man"; a young female client who wears sexy nightgowns and makeup may be criticized while an elderly woman who habitually exposes herself may be virtually ignored)

Interventions

- Make individual contacts with the client on a one-to-one basis when the client is not sexually acting out, without waiting for the client to initiate contact. *This meets the client's need for interpersonal contact and validates the client as a worthwhile person.*

- Share with the client your reactions to the behavior. *Acknowledges, rather than ignores, the client's behavior, and assists the client in identifying the consequences of his or her own behavior.*

- Set realistic and consistent limits on sexual acting-out behavior (see the section on the Manipulative Client for limiting-setting suggestions). *Limits help the client to control behavior and learn what is, and is not, acceptable.*

- Provide for the client's need for privacy. *Respecting a client's privacy will avoid dehumanization.*

- Attempt to determine the meaning of the behavior to the client and the purpose that it serves, e.g., what is the client hoping to achieve? *All behavior has meaning and can be understood. Effective interventions must be based on the meaning and purpose of the client's behavior.*

- Explore one's own and the staff's responses to the client's sexual acting-out. *Self-awareness of one's own responses to sexual acting-out behavior will increase the nurse's own comfort in dealing with these clients and will increase the likelihood that the nurse will be able to develop effective interventions.*

Communicating with the Sexually Aggressive Client

Client: After calling the nurse to his room to see a pornographic poster he has hung, James says "I thought you'd like to see my poster, and I was also hoping you'd be able to give me a back rub."

Nurse: "James, I feel uncomfortable being in your room since you hung that poster. I would appreciate it if you'd keep it in a more private place." *Rationale: Sharing the nurse's personal reaction of discomfort, while recognizing that the client can keep the poster privately, acknowledges the client's right and demonstrates that the client's behavior has consequences.*	Nurse: "This poster seems to be important to you. What's that all about?" *Rationale: This strategy is an attempt to discover the meaning the poster has for the client and what the client expects to gain from its display.*

ANGRY CLIENT

The angry client is experiencing the feeling of anger, expressing this feeling, and usually some interaction is taking place around the anger.

Assessment Cues

- Speaking in loud agitated tones; yelling, harshness, foul language, blaming and/or speaking in a menacing, low voice
- Behavioral cues such as: nostril flaring, fist clenching, pacing, glaring, jaw clenching, muttering
- Loss of control with objects could predict loss of control, and violence, toward people
- Fearful looks, refusing to talk, making threats, any change to usual behavior
- Physiological responses to stress: increased heart rate, respirations, BP; shaky knees, sweating, confusion, cold hands, sweaty palms, squeaky voice, restlessness

Interventions

- Learn to recognize this client's triggers for anger. *Individuals are disturbed and threatened by slightly different stimuli. Explore what causes anger for this client.*
- Respond to agitated and angry behaviors with support and empathy. *Your affect, especially in the initial phases of the expression of anger, helps balance the communication.*
- Respond to defensive and aggressive behaviors and communications by giving choices, setting limits, using directive statements, and being scrupulous about being non-judgmental. *This structures the encounter into a productive problem-solving mode while addressing the client's feelings.*
- If threats, violence, or loss of control are present give the client space, speak clearly and plainly, and check your body posture. *Space minimizes collateral damage, communication is more efficient, and your body must be in a position to deal with a crisis.*
- Discuss the expression of angry feelings with the client after all is resolved. *This conversation models appropriate follow-up to strong feelings and conveys messages about coping skills.*

Communicating with the Angry Client

Client: "There is no way you people are going to treat me like that! Who do you think you are? Where do you get off even thinking that I'd tolerate this?"

Nurse: "Tell me what is going on." *Rationale: Involving the client in a clear, concise communication where attention is being paid to her thoughts and feelings.*	Nurse: "How can I help you?" *Rationale: Establishes willingness to work out a solution to the problem as the client sees it.*

ANXIOUS CLIENT

Anxious people feel apprehensive or tense as a result of anticipating an imagined threat. At times they are unable to identify a specific threat.

Assessment Cues

Moderate Anxiety

- Occasional shortness of breath
- Mild gastric symptoms, such as "butterflies" in the stomach
- Facial twitches, trembling lips
- Selective inattention
- Narrowing of the perceptual field

Severe Anxiety

- Frequent shortness of breath
- Increased heart rate, possible premature contractions
- Elevated blood pressure
- Dry mouth, upset stomach, anorexia, diarrhea or constipation
- Body trembling, fearful facial expression, tense muscles, restlessness, exaggerated startle response, inability to relax, difficulty falling asleep
- Extremely narrowed perceptual field
- Difficulty problem solving or organizing

Panic

- Shortness of breath, choking or smothering sensation

- Hypotension, dizziness, chest pain or pressure, palpitations, chills or hot flashes, sweating
- Nausea
- Agitation, poor motor coordination, involuntary movements, entire body trembling, facial expression of terror
- Feeling of losing control, fear of dying
- Completely disrupted perceptual field

Children and Adolescents
- Impaired academic achievement
- Inappropriate behavior with peers, leading to dislike and isolation
- Poor self-concept

Interventions

Moderate to Severe Anxiety
- Suggest distraction techniques such as listening to music, reading a book, talking to a friend, playing a game, or counting backward by threes. *Distraction techniques allow people to remain in control when experiencing moderate levels of anxiety.*
- Suggest that they use a journal to keep track of thoughts, feelings, and memories. *This self-monitoring technique helps people identify events preceding, during and after anxiety occurs.*
- Teach muscle relaxation and deep breathing exercises and have clients practice these techniques twice a day for 20 minutes. *With practice they can recognize when their bodies are tightening up and learn how to cope with stress by deep breathing, which stops the escalation of anxiety.*
- Discuss the benefits of exercise and design a program that fits their lifestyle. Have them maintain a progress chart. *Exercise has an overall relaxing effect on the body. A progress chart may motivate adherence to the exercise program.*

Panic
- Use a calm approach and stay with individuals who are experiencing the panic level of anxiety. *Promotes safety and reduces fear.*
- Speak slowly in a gentle voice, using short, simple sentences. *People in panic level of anxiety have great difficulty focusing or concentrating.*

- Tell them to take slow, deep breaths and to imagine inhaling and exhaling through the soles of their feet. *During panic people feel disconnected from the environment and this imagery helps people feel grounded.*

Children and Adolescents

- Teach them to redefine the sensations of anxiety as sensations of excitement. *They will be less disabled by their physical and emotional experience if their expectations are positive.*

Communicating with the Anxious Client

Client: Glancing away, crossing and uncrossing her legs. "I'm sorry that I seem so anxious. I don't know what I'm supposed to say . . ."

| Nurse: "I'll just sit with you until group begins. I want to listen to whatever you would like to say, or we can just sit here quietly."
 Rationale: Responding to her worry about saying the "wrong" thing by accepting any topic with which she would like to begin. Giving permission to not talk if this is what she chooses to do. | Nurse: "It is often difficult to know where to begin. Perhaps you could tell me a little bit about yourself."
 Rationale: Normalizing her concern and sense of helplessness. Provides a general direction, at the same time giving her the control to choose what to share. |

COGNITIVELY IMPAIRED CLIENT

A cognitively impaired client is someone who has impairments in abstract thinking, judgment, insight, complex capabilities (language, tasks, recognition), and memory, and has spatial disorientation, some personality changes, and an altered effect.

Assessment Cues

- Cannot process or remember new information; can no longer follow a multistepped process to conclusion
- Misjudges distances and falls, injures self, or knocks things over
- Has difficulty recognizing everyday objects, such as a key or a pen. An otherwise quiet person talks loudly about sex
- Believes oneself to be considerably younger (i.e., a child)

- Is easily startled, or lashes out angrily, when someone approaches from the side or behind
- Interacts stiffly or angrily with family members and asks who they are

Interventions

- Minimize the loss of self-care capacity. Support the client's self-care capacity by reinforcing the use of current skills for as long as possible. *This can help to maintain a level of functioning that would otherwise deteriorate.*
- The client should be wearing whatever aids (hearing, vision) are necessary to prevent sensory loss or distortion. Be aware of sensory overload situations such as loud sounds that bounce off hard surfaces; this can distort sounds and disorient the client. *Structure the client's environment to support cognitive functions. Eliminate problematic low light.*
- Orient the client with familiar objects from home, such as slippers, robe, and photographs. *The disorientation associated with cognitive decline can be distressing. Regularly seeing something from home might focus the client.*
- Family members and caregivers must learn how to work with the client. Promote their education about the illness through professional help, support groups, and self-help groups. *Explain the disease process and the practical problems that arise from each stage of the illness. Explore coping and management strategies.*
- Behaviorally manage the client. *Respond to problems with a behavioral (rather than a pharmacological or cognitive) program of interventions. For example, an agitated client who was an engineer wants to go home with his wife. Staff ask him to help them fix a problem with a chair. He becomes involved with his project and tells his wife he'll be along later. The distraction allows the client to refocus.*
- Pharmacological interventions need to be used judiciously and have low anticholinergic impacts. *Anticholinergic effects worsen cognitive impairments. Options such as low doses of risperidone would be an improvement over conventional antipsychotics.*
- Typical sleep difficulties are worsened by confusion and aggravate the disorientation that may be experienced in lowered light. The most helpful measure may be to allow sleepless clients to wander in a safe, confined area until they are tired. *A*

hallway architecturally designed to allow safe wandering promotes mobility while allowing an expenditure of energy. A small amount of beer or wine at bedtime may produce enough relaxation without side effects if physical activity is not effective.

- If the client is disorganized at night, make sure the room is light and without shadows. Possibly leave on a radio to provide more stimulation. *Cognitively impaired clients can distort sensory input. Find a balance between turning up the volume on the radio that may help the person hear one range of sounds and causing sensory overload because the rest of the sounds are too loud.*

- Gently orient the client. To allay anxiety, do not argue with the client about verbal discrepancies. Rather, direct the client toward areas of interest that are familiar and pleasurable. *Prioritize the client's comfort and activity over total accuracy.*

Communicating with the Cognitively Impaired Client

Client: "I have to go get ready for my father. He's taking me to the zoo."

Nurse: "Would you like to wear one of these sweaters? It might get chilly later." *Rationale: Distraction to an activity without arguing or challenging the client's thinking prioritizes the activity over her ideas about her father.*	**Nurse: "I'm Eileen and I can help you get ready if you want. You have some lovely things."** *Rationale: Explaining who you are, even if the person sees you several times a day, minimizes the chance of the client having a frightening encounter with a stranger. Then having a somewhat structured social interaction sets the tone for further socialization.*

DELUSIONAL CLIENT

A delusional client is someone who holds mistaken or false beliefs about himself or the environment that are firmly held, even in the face of disconfirming evidence.

Assessment Cues

- Talks about having special powers or abilities

- Describes events with unsupported explanations
- Puts all information into the same framework
- Insists upon a particular, irrational view
- Believes global events are referring to him, such as describing a story on the radio as specifically addressed to him
- Client cannot tell the difference between the delusion ("I'm married to Nicole Kidman.") and a personal preference ("I'd love to live like a Hollywood idol.")

Interventions

- Attend seriously to the client. *This is one of the most direct and successful ways to demonstrate caring and respect for a delusional client.*
- Respond to the feeling state the client is experiencing. *Talking about the feelings a client is having helps give a common focus to the intervention and encourages the discussion of feelings in the future.*
- Reassure clients of their safety. *Having delusional thinking can be a frightening experience.*
- Monitor for the client's particular prodromal symptoms (those symptoms that occur early in the relapse process for that client). *Once identified, prompt clinical intervention with antipsychotic medication may reduce the overall frequency of the relapse event.*
- Delay or prevent relapse through treatment. *Combining maintenance antipsychotic medication therapy with psychosocial approaches has been found to be more effective than pharmacotherapy alone in treating delusional symptoms.*
- Validate reality. *Make a distinction between what is actually happening in a client's surroundings and what may be perceived because of the symptom.*
- Set realistic goals for client change. *Decide what is the most important effort to expend at this time so that valuable resources are not squandered and success is probable.*
- Focus upon the most troublesome areas of client functioning and set incremental, short-term goals that pave the way for successes in achieving long-term goals. *Clients with schizophrenia are extremely sensitive to change and failure.*

Communicating with the Delusional Client

Client: "I have to try to remove her. Her eyes moved, showing she has demon influences. It's my responsibility."

Nurse: "I hear you saying how important this is to you. Can you talk to me about what kind of pressure this puts on you?" *Rationale: Validates the emotional impact of his thinking while encouraging talking about feelings.*	Nurse: "We also have responsibilities to make sure you are thinking clearly and safely. You know you can depend on us to help you." *Rationale: Accentuates the available support from others, the need to think and talk before acting, and the need for treatment.*

DEMANDING CLIENT

A demanding client gets needs met through a style of interacting that places burdens upon others expecting that others will provide for the client.

Assessment Cues

- The client makes demands of others rather than requests
- Demanding statements begin with "you," such as "You better give me what I want"
- Cues of the client's impacts on others are not responded to by the demanding client
- Demands are made in an impatient, harsh tone
- There is no recognition or caring that the demand places a strain or an unreasonable difficulty on others
- The client may have an inability to cope with negative responses to requests or an underlying fear of making requests

Interventions

- Assess the likely outcome of your interactions. *If the client's demands escalate, comply within reason and discuss the matter later when the client is not agitated.*
- Ask the client to express needs, as opposed to making demand. *This helps the client make a distinction between stating a need and making a demand.*
- Teach alternative interactions. *Proper communication styles may not occur naturally and have to be taught.*

- Discuss in detail the way in which the client is talking to others, and focus less on what he is actually demanding. *Focusing on the tone of the message, rather than the objects or experiences, reinforces the importance of being mindful of interactions.*

- Explore why the client feels it necessary to demand rather than request. *There may be psychodynamic reasons why this particular mode of discourse has been reinforced for this client.*

- Do not become demoralized by incessant demands. *Make sure the boundaries between you the client are intact so that you are not absorbing the emotional whirlwind that demanding clients can create.*

Communicating with the Demanding Client

Client: "You better give that to me right now if you know what's good for you."

Nurse: "I'd be happy to give that to you. And could you give me 5 minutes to talk later on?" *Rationale: This response would be appropriate to defuse a situation and discuss the demanding style when the client is not stressed by a need.*	Nurse: "I understand that there is something you want right now. It sounds like it's important to you." *Rationale: Giving recognition and reflecting feelings validates the client's concerns.*

DEPENDENT CLIENT

The dependent person has a pervasive and excessive need to be taken care of. This need leads to clinging and submissive behaviors.

Assessment Cues

- Inability to make decisions or function independently
- Demonstrates clinging and ingratiating behaviors
- Passively accepts the leadership of others
- Fearful of separation
- Views self as helpless
- Seeks out dominant others to lean on for guidance, control, support and permission

- Experiences anxiety when the dominant other is unavailable
- Difficulty in initiating projects
- Functions adequately only when assured of approval and supervision
- Subordinates desires and needs to the wishes of others in order to maintain the relationship
- May have several other DSM-IV-TR Axis II diagnoses
- Is often responded to with anger and resentment because of continuous clinging and ingratiating behaviors

Interventions

- Encourage client to perform self-care activities. *This fosters independent living skills.*
- Avoid doing for the client those things the client is capable of doing without help and set realistic limits on what should, and should not, be done for the client. *This strategy promotes independence by minimizing the client's dependence on others.*
- Schedule regular sessions as a way to anticipate client needs before the client demands attention through inappropriate responses. *Anticipatory guidance will minimize the client's anxiety and thus reduce acting out.*
- Help the client identify assets and liabilities, including plans for change; emphasize client strengths and potentials. *Self-assessment can enhance a positive self-concept.*
- Encourage the client to take responsibility for the client's own opinions and point out when the client negates his or her own feelings or opinions. *Taking responsibility fosters independence and enhances self-esteem.*
- Encourage the client to recognize the choices the client has in terms of behavior. *Recognizing personal responsibility and choices of behavior further optimizes independent functioning.*
- Share with the client your observations of the client's dependent behavior. *Feedback from staff and peers fosters self-awareness.*
- Explore with the client the consequences of the client's behavior—that is, clinging tends to result in avoidance by others. *Recognizing the relationship between what one does and how others respond forms the rationale for behavioral change.*
- Give positive reinforcement for successful achievements. *Recognizing the ability to succeed validates the client's independence and encourages further behavioral change.*

Communicating with the Dependent Client

Client: Said desperately, "You must help me right now! It's too hard for me to do this by myself."

Nurse: "Nancy, in the past you've been capable of making appointments on your own. Let's see you do this now." *Rationale: Pointing out previous success reinforces the client's sense of mastery. Encouraging the client to do what she is capable of doing encourages independence.*	Nurse: "Asking for help with tasks that you can do for yourself will cause others to leave you alone. It's more effective to ask for help only with tasks that are really difficult for you." *Rationale: Confronting the client with the consequences of her clinging, demanding behavior encourages her to evaluate her choices.*

DEPRESSED CLIENT

People who are depressed experience a loss of interest in life, a dejected mood, negative thinking, and slowed physiological processes. Many clients have recurrent episodes.

Assessment Cues

- Decreased desire to participate in activities or interact with other people
- Increased dependency on others
- Mood is one of despair or desolation
- Feelings of guilt
- Frequent crying or the inability to cry
- Focuses on failures, sees self as incompetent, catastrophizes, harshly critical of self
- Believes present and future are hopeless, anticipates disapproval from others
- Decreased ability to make decisions
- Decrease in rate and number of thoughts
- Believes self to be unattractive or ugly
- In psychotic depression, delusions and hallucinations may be present
- Loss of sexual desire
- Appetite increased or decreased in early stages; decreased in severe depression

- Sleep more or less in early stages; decreased sleep in severe depression
- Psychomotor retardation
- Constipation
- Unkempt, poor hygiene

Interventions

- Assess for suicidal thoughts and plans. *The first priority of care is client safety. Since as many as 15% of clients who are depressed commit suicide, it is critical that you determine suicide potential.* (See Suicidal Client for further information.)

- Help clients identify repetitive statements that are self-negative. Point out examples of dysfunctional thinking as it occurs. *The purpose is to help clients understand that negative thinking is a symptom of depression, not necessarily fact.*

- Give clients plenty of time to respond verbally to your questions. *Since their thought processes are slowed down, they need more time to respond. Answering for them gives the message that you view them as incapable and is a blow to their self-esteem.*

- Encourage clients to participate in activities with one person to begin, adding more people to the group as time goes on. Help them identify the benefits of social interactions. *The more alone and isolated people are, the more depressed they feel.*

- If client and partner introduce their concerns about sexual disinterest, explain that desire usually returns as the depression lifts. *Understanding that desire is a symptom of depression will decrease feelings of hurt, inadequacy, and guilt. Identifying benefits reinforces positive behavioral change.*

- If decision-making is a problem, provide limited choices until their abilities improve. *This will increase self-confidence and self-esteem and allows as much control as they can manage effectively.*

- Explore clients' previous successes, encouraging them to identify their own strengths and abilities. *This reinforces previous positive coping skills.*

- Help them clarify what they need and want by setting clear goals and facilitating their identification of resources. *As they begin to advocate for themselves, they will become more hopeful and self-sufficient.*

- Use reality testing to help clients identify possible irrational beliefs. *Global statements about guilt and inadequacy contribute to low self-esteem.*

- Help clients choose recreational activities that are consistent with their physical, emotional, and social capabilities. In the acute phase, keep activities simple and short. *People who are depressed often forget to do the things that make them feel better. They have a limited attention span and ability to concentrate.*

- Set limits on the amount of time clients spend discussing past failures. *Rumination intensifies guilt and low self-esteem.*

- Help client design positive self-statements and repeat these several times a day. Review their past joys and successes in life. *Positive thoughts and expectations increase self-esteem. Having purpose and joy in life is a component of spirituality.*

- Encourage behaviors that foster an internal locus of control. *Feelings of control counteract the feelings of helplessness that are part of depression.*

- Facilitate client's use of meditation, prayer, and other spiritual and religious traditions. *For many people religious beliefs improve self-esteem, life satisfaction, and the ability to cope.*

- Assess how the family's behavior affects the client and how the client's behavior affects the family. Discuss how family strengths and resources can be used to enhance the health status of the client and the family's ability to cope. *Mood disorders not only affect clients but also their family and friends. You must consider all significant others to be recipients of your care.*

Communicating with the Depressed Client

Client: Looking down at her hands in her lap, shoulders slumped. "I've been very sad since Christmas time."

Nurse: "Are you aware of anything happening about that time that triggered your feeling of sadness?" *Rationale: Assessing for a particular event that may have contributed to her depression. This information might give direction to nursing interventions such as grieving, anger management, or self-esteem issues.*	Nurse: "That's a long time. It must be very difficult to feel that down for so long." *Rationale: Acknowledging her feelings of depression. Responding with empathy for her struggle.*

EATING-DISORDERED CLIENT

People with eating disorders are preoccupied with their body image and view dieting or purging as the solution to all of their problems.

Assessment Cues

Anorexia

- Overcompliant
- Obsessive rituals concerning eating and exercise
- Refusal to eat may be a way to gain control or power in the family
- Presence of a secondary food phobia
- Presence of multiple fears
- Cognitive distortions include selective abstraction, overgeneralization, magnification, ideas of reference, superstitious thinking, and dichotomous thinking
- Severely distorted body image that often reaches delusional proportions
- Perfectionistic standards for self
- Social withdrawal
- Decreased blood volume contributing to hypotension, decreased blood flow to the kidneys, decreased cardiac chamber dimensions, and decreased cardiac output
- Amenorrhea related to stress, percentage of body fat lost, and altered hypothalamic function
- Osteoporosis
- Weight loss of 25 to 50 percent of normal weight

Bulimia

- Cyclic behavioral pattern of dieting or fasting, binge eating, and purging the body of ingested food
- Sporadic excessive exercise
- Repression of feelings and avoiding conflict to protect from anticipated rejection
- Multiple fears and a sense of hopelessness
- Great concern about not regaining the weight they lose
- Believe that if they could only be thin, all other problems would be solved

- Perfectionistic standards for self
- Social withdrawal
- Electrolyte imbalance causing muscle weakness, seizures, arrhythmias, and even death
- GI complications such as constipation, cathartic colon, and laxative dependence
- Frequent vomiting leads to esophagitis, perforation of the esophagus, decreased tooth enamel, chronic sore throat, and swollen salivary glands
- Weight may be within normal range

Interventions

- Use the term weight restoration. *The term weight gain often creates an instant phobic response.*
- Identify a reasonable target weight with a range of four to six pounds. *Reassures clients that they will not be forced to become overweight. The range helps them learn to accept a certain amount of normal weight fluctuation.*
- Negotiate a reasonable contract for amounts to be eaten for each meal and snack. *The sensation of bloating may lessen if the calories are spread across six meals a day.*
- Physical activity should be adapted to the client's food intake and with consideration of bone mineral density and cardiac function. *The focus is on helping clients assume responsibility for themselves as they move from the destructive use of exercise to healthy exercise.*
- Help clients identify secondary gains. *Accurate identification leads to effective interventions. Needs will be met in constructive and healthy ways.*
- Help them identify underlying fears and negative emotions. *Misinterpretation of emotions with sensations of hunger contributes to binge eating.*
- Encourage clients to keep a food diary to record all food eaten, as well as any binge eating and purging. *This helps them analyze which particular foods and situations trigger binge eating.*
- Explore alternative coping behaviors. *Insight into high-risk situations will help clients gain control of binges.*
- Teach clients and families that it is the client who needs to take responsibility for her or his own eating behavior. *Conflict about food is likely to be counterproductive.*

Communicating with the Eating-Disordered Client

Client: "This hospital took away my rights. It happens at home too. You'd think I'd be used to it by now, but I get so angry that I don't know what to do."

Nurse: "How are your rights taken away at home?" *Rationale: Seeking clarification. Comparing and contrasting the hospital with the home environment may help client gain insight into behavior that triggers a response from others.*	**Nurse: "What do you do with your anger when you feel this out of control?"** *Rationale: Assessing for effectiveness of usual coping patterns. First step in the problem-solving process.*

FEARFUL CLIENT

Some people are fearful of others and are often referred to as being extremely shy.

Assessment Cues

- Overly sensitive to the opinions of others
- Easily hurt by criticism
- Devastated by the slightest hint of disapproval
- Exaggerated need for acceptance
- Terrified of being embarrassed
- Reluctant to enter into relationships without a guarantee of unconditional approval
- Fear rejection and abandonment
- Lack self-confidence

Interventions

- Your approach should be one of self-determination. *Clients are partners in treatment and have the right to choose their own course in life.*
- The focus is on role functioning. *Recognize that not all fear or shyness will disappear. Clients need to adapt as best they can.*
- Help clients maintain hope. *Fearful people are particularly susceptible to loss of hope for change and giving up on treatment.*
- Communicate to clients that you recognize their feelings of helplessness and fears of becoming more independent. *This*

expression of empathy will help them be more collaborative in the problem-solving process.

- If client views you as an all-powerful person who will make everything better, avoid rescuing behaviors. *If you rescue the client it reinforces the feeling of helplessness and the external locus of control.*

- Help clients identify what would be different, what they would gain, and what they would lose if they were less fearful. *As they identify what they would like out of particular situations, they can problem solve ways to achieve their goal.*

- Encourage and support interactions with others. *Never force interaction when clients need to maintain their distance.*

- Provide social skills training and assertiveness training. *This helps them identify interpersonal problems resulting from social skill deficits and use specific skills to overcome deficits.*

- Role-play and provide feedback about the appropriateness of their responses. *This encourages them to evaluate their behavior in social situations.*

- Involve clients in group therapy. *Group therapy is one way to develop and foster better relationships with others, decrease isolation, and increase the sense of feeling understood.*

- Encourage clients to make their own decisions. *This reinforces a sense of competence and an internal locus of control.*

- Discuss their abilities and limitations. *This promotes realistic self-appraisal.*

Communicating with the Fearful Client

Client: "There is this girl in my philosophy class who I really admire. I would like to ask her out, but she will probably say no. I've never even said hello to her."

Nurse: "Let's think about the steps leading up to asking her out. What do you think the first step might be?" *Rationale: Teaching the use of the problem-solving process and planning one small step at a time may lessen the overwhelming fear of rejection.*	**Nurse:** "Let's role play this situation. I'll be you and you be the girl in the class." *Rationale: Role-playing is an effective intervention in decreasing fear and increasing a sense of capability. By taking the role of the client first, the nurse can model appropriate social interaction.*

GRIEVING CLIENT

Grieving is the reaction to an actual or impending loss such as the death of a loved one, or the loss of an object or situation that has a part in defining a person's self-worth (the loss of another's love, the loss of a job, the loss of a pet, the loss of physical functioning, the loss of self-esteem, loss of status, financial disaster, etc.). Grief reactions may be uncomplicated (one in which the individual is able to face the reality of the loss and is immersed in the work of grieving), or dysfunctional (grieving may be delayed or rejected, or the length or extent of symptoms extend beyond the usual in intensity or length and interfere with the resolution of grief).

Assessment Cues

- The duration and expression of "normal" grieving vary considerably among different cultural groups. Know what is "normal" for the individual's culture before labeling grieving as abnormal

- Look for evidence of uncomplicated grief reaction—sadness, crying, insomnia, poor appetite, weight loss, decreased interest in social activities, thinking that one hears the voice of, or transiently sees the image of, the deceased person

- If the symptoms remain present to the same extent two months after the loss, assess the individual for the possibility of major depressive disorder

- Identify any factors that may place the person at high risk for a complicated or dysfunctional grief reaction. These include an inability to share the loss with others; lack of social recognition for the loss (e.g., social recognition may be limited if the death is the result of an accidental drug overdose, suicide, or AIDS); an ambivalent relationship with the deceased; guilt about actions taken or not taken by the survivor around the time of death; traumatic circumstances surrounding the death; concurrent life crises at the time of the loss

- Assess for the presence of dysfunctional grieving—the duration of the grieving may be prolonged beyond the usual period, or the person has symptoms that are not characteristic of a "normal" grief reaction (e.g., morbid preoccupation with worthlessness, marked psychomotor retardation, thoughts of suicide, hallucinatory experiences

Interventions

- Encourage the person to talk about the actual or impending loss and acknowledge the loss. *Acknowledging the loss is the first step in grief resolution and anticipatory grieving.*

- Help the person to identify and express feelings about the loss in an atmosphere of understanding, relatedness and acceptance. *Validating the person's feelings and the person's right to express these feelings facilitates the grieving process.*

- Join with the bereaved person in a therapeutic grief ritual that may be a part of the person's cultural or religious heritage and/or arrange for pastoral counseling if the individual wishes it. *Spiritual support gives comfort and helps the person to resolve grief.*

- Remind the bereaved that they need time to grieve, and that people grieve at their own pace. *Although the grieving process takes an average of 18 months for most people, it is perfectly natural and normal for the period to be either shorter or longer. Knowing that one will eventually feel better is comforting and instills hope.*

- Identify for the bereaved the normal behaviors associated with grieving—distractibility, forgetfulness, rumination about the deceased, preoccupation with own health, and mood swings. *Interpreting this behavior as normal is supportive and consoling. Recognizing the broad spectrum of human responses to loss supports the individual's right to mourn in his or her own way.*

- Explore the effectiveness and adaptability of the bereaved person's defenses and coping mechanisms. *Helping the individual to identify strengths and effective coping mechanisms encourages self-awareness and provides the individual with specific methods to use in coping with the loss.*

- Point out the maladaptive nature of any negative or self-destructive strategies. *This strategy helps the individual to explore more adaptive means of coping.*

- If a complicated or dysfunctional grief response is present, refer the person to appropriate resources—anger management, guilt work facilitation, forgiveness facilitation, individual or family therapy—when the problems are beyond one's scope of practice. *Pathologic grief responses can be very complicated, do not usually remit by themselves, and require the help of an experienced clinician.*

- Encourage the person to join a bereavement group, try relaxation therapy methods, or seek help on an individual basis or in family therapy during critical periods. *People experiencing a loss generally find bereavement groups very helpful. A bereaved person may need special support around holiday periods or the anniversary of the death (one month, six months, one year).*

Communicating with the Grieving Client

Client: "I've been so lonely since Joe passed away. We did everything together. He was my best friend."

Nurse: "Tell me what a typical day's been like for you since Joe died." *Rationale: Asking what a typical day has been like accomplishes two goals—gathering data for assessment of the level of the client's adaptation to the loss and demonstrating interest in her.*	Nurse: "It's hard to be without your best friend. I know they can't substitute for Joe, but, who are your other friends?" *Rationale: Empathizing with the client and exploring the extent of her support system.*

HALLUCINATING CLIENT

A client who hallucinates experiences sensations that are not real in one of the five senses: hearing (the most common), seeing, smelling, tasting, and touching.

Assessment Cues

Auditory

- Moving eyes back and forth as if looking for someone
- Listening intently to a person who is not speaking
- Engaging in conversation with an invisible person
- Grinning or laughter that seems inappropriate
- Slowed verbal responses as if preoccupied

Visual

- Suddenly appearing startled, frightened, or terrified by another person or object or by no apparent stimulus
- Suddenly running into another room

Olfactory
- Wrinkling nose as if smelling something horrible
- Smelling parts of the body
- Smelling the air while walking toward another person
- Responding to an odor with terror

Tactile
- Slapping self as if putting out a fire
- Trying to push invisible things, like bugs, off the body

Gustatory
- Complaining about the taste of food
- Describing a bad taste without having eaten
- Spitting or scraping tongue to remove an offensive flavor

Interventions

- Use one-to-one interactions to shape and guide the situation. *Individual contact is more manageable and makes it easier to communicate for the hallucinating client.*
- Reduce excess noise and distractions. One person speaks to the client at a time. *Hallucinations can be distracting and intrusive. Keep the stimulus to a minimum.*
- Attend seriously to the client and to what the client says. *This is one of the most direct and successful ways to demonstrate caring and respect for a client who is hallucinating.*
- When the client is responding to hallucinations, address the emotion instead of the content. For example, if the client is frightened because she sees children fighting in her room, reassure. Say, "You are in a safe place." *The client's feeling, and not what that feeling is about, can be talked about without arguing about whether there are children in her room.*
- Assure that the client's room has some stimulation, to help the client block out hallucinations and support reality testing. *Isolation contributes to disorientation and distorted perceptions.*
- Respond to the feeling. *Talking about the feeling associated with the hallucinations helps give a common focus to the intervention and encourages the discussion of feelings in the future.*
- Monitor for the client's particular prodromal symptoms (those symptoms that occur early in the relapse process for that client). *Once identified, prompt clinical intervention with antipsychotic medication may reduce the overall frequency of the relapse event.*

- Delay or prevent relapse through treatment. *Combining maintenance antipsychotic medication therapy with psychosocial approaches has been found to be more effective than pharmacotherapy alone in treating hallucinatory symptoms.*

Communicating with the Hallucinating Client

Client: "I am a hungry, hungry snake. See how my scales overlap and shine?"

Nurse: "I hear you saying you are hungry. Would you like to have something to eat?"	Nurse: "Can you talk to me about what is going on for you right now?"
Rationale: Validate the statement about being hungry without invalidating the client's experience of seeing his body covered in shiny, overlapping scales.	*Rationale: This intervention helps you determine the extent and nature of the client's hallucinations. It also defines you as a caring professional who is willing to discuss his experiences.*

MANIC CLIENT

People in the manic phase of bipolar disorder have extremes of emotion which alternate with normal or depressed mood.

Assessment Cues

- Interested in all activities—constantly seeking fun and excitement; talkative and gregarious in interactions with others
- Forms intense attachments rapidly
- Feels independent and self-sufficient
- Mood is unstable: euphoric and irritable
- Unable to experience feelings of guilt
- May have brief episodes of crying
- Grandiose beliefs about self
- Inordinate positive expectations; unable to see potential negative outcomes
- Irate if criticized by others
- Flight of ideas
- Believes self to be unusually beautiful or handsome
- Delusions of grandeur; some may experience hallucinations
- Increase in sexual activity and partners
- Difficulty eating due to inability to sit still

- Sleeps only one or two hours a night
- Hyperactive motor behavior
- Constipation
- Frequent changes of clothing; prefers bright clothing

Interventions

- If the environment is overstimulating, redirect or remove clients to a quieter place. Suggest that they avoid stimulating places such as bars or busy shopping malls. *People in a manic state may become exhausted when excessive levels of activity are combined with decreased awareness of fatigue.*

- Set limits on intrusive or interruptive behaviors. Teach and reinforce social roles and the appropriate expression of feelings. *Because they are interested in every person and every activity in the environment, they may be very intrusive in other people's conversations and activities and create socially awkward situations.*

- If clients are experiencing flight of ideas, decrease environmental stimuli. Listen for unexpressed messages and feelings as well as the overt content of the conversation. *Active listening and feedback will improve their efforts to communicate.*

- Provide impulse control training:
  1. Help them identify situations that require thoughtful action
  2. Teach them to cue themselves to "stop and think" before acting impulsively.
  3. Identify other courses of action and the predicted consequences. *This will to help them protect themselves from impulsive behavior, which could be dangerous to themselves or others.*

- Help clients develop a chart that identifies symptoms that indicate the beginning of a relapse. Plan appropriate action to take in the event of these symptoms. *It is easier to manage mood instability before the episode has cycled into a manic phase.*

- Help clients choose recreational activities that are consistent with their physical, emotional, and social capabilities. In the acute phase, keep activities simple and short. *People in the manic phase are interested in every activity, whether appropriate or not. Their attention span is very short, due to distractibility.*

- Do not argue about their delusions. *You do not want to put them in the position of having to defend their belief.*

- Facilitate their use of meditation, prayer, and other spiritual or religious traditions. *For many people religious beliefs improve self-esteem, life satisfaction, and the ability to cope.*

- Assess how the family's behavior affects the client and how the client's behavior affects the family. Discuss how family strengths and resources can be used to enhance the health status of the client and the family's ability to cope. *Mood disorders not only affect clients, but their family and friends. You must consider all significant others to be recipients of your care.*

- Meals should be eaten in a quiet environment. *Too many distractions will interfere with nutritional intake.*

- Provide high-calorie foods that can be eaten while walking or moving about. Intake must be sufficient to provide energy for their high activity level. *Since it is difficult to sit still for more than a few minutes, they may eat more if they can move about at the same time.*

Communicating with the Manic Client

Client: "I can't find anyone to love me. No one ever chose me. I once found someone to love me. She was 21. (Begins crying.) Her name was Tiffany, but I lost her phone number. Now she is out there waiting for me."

Nurse: "You sound so very lonely and abandoned." *Rationale: Reflecting back his feelings. Letting him know that you hear him, understand, and care about how he feels.*	**Nurse: "It sounds like you think there is no hope for a relationship for you. Is that a realistic belief?"** *Rationale: A cognitive approach to help client evaluate thoughts realistically.*

MANIPULATIVE CLIENT

A manipulative person exploits other people and situations for personal gain. Learning to meet one's needs directly is the major challenge for those who demonstrate manipulative behavior.

Assessment Cues

Nonverbal

- Smiling to excess

- Touching others inappropriately
- Crying, whining in public
- Appearing confused and helpless
- Drawing attention to self (falling, dramatic displays of somatic problems)
- Giving gifts to others
- Tardiness for appointments
- Selective forgetting
- Refusing to participate in activities or treatment program
- Seductive dressing, eye movements, body language
- Decreased tolerance for frustration
- Self/other destructive acting-out

Verbal

- Compliments or flatters others
- Sarcasm
- Threats
- Demanding behavior
- Inducing guilt in others ("I thought we had a relationship of trust.")
- Excessive criticism of others
- Bargaining for special privileges
- Being overly solicitous of others
- Wanting to be exempt from rules ("Couldn't I have my medication just one hour earlier?")
- Mimicking the therapeutic responses used by staff members ("I have a feeling you're angry with me.")
- Playing one staff member against another (splitting)
- Confronting staff in the presence of other clients
- Lying
- Telling the nurse what he or she "wants" to hear
- Using information about others to exploit them
- Excessive involvement in the problems of others
- Aggressive questioning about personal matters
- Rationalizing, projecting, and minimizing blame for own behavior
- Self-pity
- Role reversal

Interventions

- Develop a team approach to the client, but assign one staff member as a primary resource person. *Consistency prevents opportunities for splitting the staff.*

- Set realistic limits (consistent expectations and guidelines for self-control) with enforceable consequences on the behavior that is most dysfunctional and problematic. *If limits are imposed unrealistically or globally, the client will only be more likely to rebel and the dysfunctional behavior will escalate. Unpleasant consequences may help decrease negative behavior.*

- Share with the client the reasons for limits and consequences of violating the limits. *The client can make appropriate choices when in possession of complete information.*

- Model respect, honesty, openness, and assertiveness. *Modeling demonstrates expected behavior and enhances the client's learning.*

- Interact with client when the client is not acting out. *This strategy reinforces positive behavior.*

- Confront the client each time manipulation occurs. *Consequences must follow behavior closely in order to be effective.*

- Discuss with the client alternative ways of dealing with people and situations. *This strategy promotes personal responsibility.*

- Help client identify assets. *Identifying assets focuses on positive behavior and promotes self-esteem.*

- Remove limits from treatment plan when the client adheres to objectives consistently. *Removing limits under this condition rewards appropriate behavior.*

- Evaluate effectiveness of limit setting. Limit setting may have to be altered for greater effectiveness. *Evaluation also helps to clarify discharge planning goals.*

- Jointly develop contracts for behavioral change. *Collaboration with the client in the client's treatment plan establishes client responsibility.*

- Teach stress-reduction techniques (guided imagery, relaxation) and cognitive techniques (thought stopping). *Alternative measures defuse anxiety and reinforce the ability for self-control.*

- Involve client in assertiveness training and problem solving. *Assertiveness training and problem-solving teach assertion, rather than aggression, as appropriate responses to people and situations.*

- Offer support to other clients who may be targets of manipulation. *Support ensures the well-being of all clients.*

Communicating with the Manipulative Client

Client: "You're the sweetest nurse on the unit. I know you can help me get a pass for next Friday."

Nurse: "Darlene, whenever you compliment me you usually want something from me." *Rationale: Confronting the client about her manipulative behavior will help her identify maladaptive approaches to others. If the nurse fails to confront the behavior consistently, the client will assume the behavior is tolerated and acceptable.*	Nurse: "Darlene, when you compliment people because you want something from them, they are not likely to trust anything you say." *Rationale: This response points out the negative consequences of the manipulative behavior. It also encourages the client to consider other ways of interacting.*

REPETITIVE AND RUMINATIVE CLIENT

The ruminative client is preoccupied with a single idea or a set of thoughts and repeats sentences, or stays fixated on a particular topic, to the exclusion of other thoughts and topics.

Assessment Cues

- Unable to talk about or think about other topics easily, at all, or for any significant length of time
- Conversations on any subject consistently return to the same theme or set of thoughts
- Restates the same set of thoughts or words in a recurring fashion
- May misperceive others' statements as referring to the same material.
- Assess for damage to frontal lobe executive functioning
- Assess ability to attend to another topic, and verbally prioritize
- Assess anxiety level if she/he does speak about other areas

Interventions

- Develop a treatment plan where reminders and cues about the content of conversations are given regularly. *This helps the clients steer contacts with others into more desirable channels.*

- Cooperatively develop a list of topics clients can use to shift conversation. *This intervention shapes clients' conversations in a way they understand and want as well as offering guidance and direction to clients.*

- Remind and prompt client about these listed topics. *This is a positive prompt and is effective when delivered more than twice prior to a negative prompt (an example of a negative prompt would be, "Remember, we agreed you'd stop talking about that.").*

- Behavioral interventions may be useful in reinforcing adaptive interactions. *Giving clients a desired experience or object when not repeating themselves connects the enjoyable with the adaptive.*

- When clients says something in a repetitive style, label that you are rephrasing their statements. *Rephrasing in this way models how the statement can be made without being repetitive.*

- Monitor your affect when communicating with repetitive clients to make sure you are not conveying impatience, frustration, or general disapproval. *Rumination is difficult for clients to minimize or extinguish and your support is necessary.*

Communicating with the Repetitive and Ruminative Client

Client: "I'm in hell with the demons. I'm in hell with the demons. I'm in hell with the demons."

Nurse: "I hear you are very upset right now. Can you tell me about that using different words?" *Rationale: Validates the emotional tone of the communication while encouraging the client to describe and expand his experience.*	Nurse: "Tell me about being mad at someone by using the words we agreed on." *Rationale: Focuses the client on one of the more adaptive ways of expressing distress or concern.*

SELF-MUTILATING CLIENT

Clients who self-mutilate deliberately destroy body tissue without conscious intent of suicide.

Assessment Cues

- Females at higher risk than males
- Rate is 30 times higher than the rate of suicide attempts
- Typically begins in adolescence
- Affects people of all ethnic backgrounds
- May occur once or sporadically, or it may become repetitive
- As many as 24 to 40 percent of mental health clients self-mutilate
- Superficial to moderate self-mutilation behaviors
    1. Skin cutting
    2. Skin carving (words, designs, symbols)
    3. Skin burning
    4. Severe skin scratching
    5. Needle sticking
    6. Self-hitting
    7. Tearing out hair
    8. Inserting dangerous objects into the vagina or rectum
    9. Ingesting sharp objects
    10. Bone breaking
    11. Interfering with wound healing
- Severe self-mutilation behaviors
    1. Eye enucleation
    2. Castration
    3. Amputation of fingers, toes, or limbs
- Stereotypic self-mutilation behaviors
    1. Head banging
    2. Finger biting
    3. Most often occurs in people who are institutionalized for cognitive impairment

Interventions

- Establish a trusting relationship. *Clients have probably experienced much criticism and little understanding regarding their self-injurious behavior.*

- Avoid scolding or shaming self-mutilating clients. *The failure to stop the self-harm leads to even greater shame and concealment.*

- Set limits to minimize the potential for physical injury. Ensure that they receive medical attention as necessary. *The goal is to keep the client as safe as possible.*

- Encourage communication about self-injury. *Clients are often secretive and shameful about the behaviors. Supportive listening may help them feel less isolated.*

- Find alternative to self-harming behaviors. *The goal is to diminish or extinguish the use of self-mutilation.*

    1. Symbolic enactments, such as drawing the "blood" or "cuts" on paper or "injuring" a toy or stuffed animal.

    2. Physical awareness activities, such as slow breathing and relaxation exercises.

    3. Distraction, such as contracting to wait 5 to 10 minutes before self-injuring, exercising, or going to a movie.

    4. Interpersonal contact, such as calling a friend or a support group member.

    5. Art and writing activities, such as drawing the feeling or the memory or writing a letter to a significant person.

    6. Expressive anger activities, such as pounding a tennis racket on a bed, pounding pillows, throwing ice cubes, or smashing aluminum cans.

Communicating with a Self-mutilating Client

Client: "It gets to the point that I feel numb inside and cutting makes me feel alive. I hate crying so now the blood has become my tears."

Nurse: "I understand the feeling of numbness. What other ways besides cutting have you tried to deal with this?" *Rationale: The first step of the problem-solving process is to determine what other measures the client has tried.*	Nurse: "That seems very symbolic, red tears. Can you tell me more about how this helps you?" *Rationale: It is important to understand the unique meaning of the behavior. Only when the meaning is understood can nursing interventions be designed.*

SLEEP-DISORDERED CLIENT

A client with a sleep disorder may be sleeping too much, too little, waiting a long time to fall asleep (sleep latency), waking up very early (early morning awakening), or have frequent awakenings during the night.

Assessment Cues

- Change in mood, including irritability or apathy
- Does not feel rested upon awakening
- Symptoms of depression may correspond with a sleep disorder
- Reports "light" sleep or "restless" sleeping
- Monitor all phases of sleep process by tracking sleep through a sleep log or other device
- Assess the sleep environment to assure reasonable conditions that enhance sleep
- Determine what was considered normal for the client, including how long it usually took to fall asleep, best bedtime, amount of restful sleep, time to wake up, conditions of sleep such as temperature, darkness, surface, covers, pillows, and ambient sound

Interventions

- Discuss sleep hygiene and the client's understanding of comfort, timing, and behaviors. *Use of stimulants such as chocolate and other caffeinated substances, the hours the client is scheduling rest, and the particulars of the sleeping area can all affect sleep.*
- Assure a consistent schedule and a reasonable sleep environment for the client. *Mental disability or circumstances may have impacted negatively on the sleep environment.*
- Educate and encourage. *Give information about sleep and what can be done to take control of the situation. This instills hope and reassurance.*
- Pharmacological interventions can be most effective when kept short term. *Dependence upon an external sleep aid such as a supplement or pharmaceutical has long-term negative consequences for sleep health.*

- Expose the client to natural sunlight or light therapy in the morning and encourage walking outdoors. *If the client is hyper-somnic, these interventions can help establish a healthier schedule.*

Communicating with a Sleep-Disordered Client

Client: "I can't get any good sleep lately. I toss and turn."

Nurse: "What time do you lie down in bed and turn the light out to go to sleep?" *Rationale: This question starts the assessment of the actual sleep conditions and schedule.*	Nurse: "How many days have you not been feeling rested when you wake up?" *Rationale: Establishes the client's conception of the chronology of the problem.*

SPIRITUALLY DISTRESSED CLIENT

Spiritual distress may include questions about values, which may or may not be related to organized religion, the loss or questioning of faith, or problems associated with converting to a new faith. In a broader sense, spiritual distress is related to fear, anger, greed, guilt, and worry.

Assessment Cues
- Struggling with the meaning and purpose of life and death
- Lack of development of moral values
- Lack of a basic sense of identity
- Feeling disconnected from family or friends
- No sense of an external power, often identified as God or a Supreme Being
- Lack of respect and acceptance of others
- No sense of fairness and justice to all members of society
- No sense of compassion for others

Interventions
- The spiritual component of the nurse–client relationship is the feeling of connection between you and the client. *Responding to the person's spirit behind the mask of their mental illness is what allows us to connect to them.*

- Respond to the whole person, who is at once spirit, mind, and body. *Both mental illness and the associated stigma eat away at people's spirits and they often feel beaten and broken. They are entitled to dignified and meaningful lives.*

- Respect the client's cultural values and religious views. *Spirituality is what allows us to connect with clients who may be very different from ourselves.*

- Allow clients to express important spiritual needs, such as the need for meaning in life, belief in God, or relief from fear, doubt, or loneliness. *It is important to recognize that spiritual needs are as diverse as our clients, their cultures, and their illnesses.*

- Foster family attitudes such as love, forgiveness, hopefulness, and acceptance. *Supporting individuals and families who seek ways to heal and achieve balance in their lives is an important aspect of spiritual nursing care.*

- Help "patients" stop being patients and instead become active consumers and collaborators. *Consumers have the right to the fullest possible control over their own lives and should be actively involved in treatment-planning decisions.*

- Explore clients' perceived lack of control over life events. *People who experience severe traumatic events often suffer from spiritual distress because the world has become threatening.*

- Support spiritual recovery for those who are victims and survivors of abuse and violence. *Their sense of purpose in life is often disrupted, as well as a loss of faith in a divine being and in other people.*

Communicating with a Spiritually Distressed Client

Client: "Why did my father abuse me? Am I some evil person who deserved to be abused?"

Nurse: "You are not responsible for, nor did you deserve, the abuse. Your father is 100 percent responsible" *Rationale: To recover from the abuse, survivors must place responsibility for the abuse where it belongs. If they fail to do this, they will continue to be paralyzed by self-blame and guilt.*	**Nurse:** "Is there something that your father did or said to you that is contributing to your sense of self-blame?" *Rationale: Perpetrators often blame the victim to escape accountability. Recognition of this attempt to deny or minimize the abusive behavior may help the survivor move past the self-blame and guilt.*

- If appropriate, refer clients to a religious counselor of their choice and support their use of prayer, or other religious traditions and rituals. *Although spirituality is not a religion, being involved in a particular religion is a way some people enhance their spirituality.*

SUBSTANCE-USING CLIENT: IN WITHDRAWAL

Withdrawal comprises the uncomfortable and maladaptive physiologic and cognitive behavioral changes that are associated with lowered blood or tissue concentrations of a substance after an individual has been engaged in heavy use of that substance.

Assessment Cues

Alcohol Withdrawal

- All except for 13.1 % of alcohol-dependent clients show physiological signs of withdrawal (Schneider, Levenson & Schnoll, 2001)
- Mild withdrawal may begin within 6–12 hours following the last drink. Symptoms may last 48–72 hours
- The appearance of hallucinations and seizures marks the onset of a major withdrawal. Major withdrawal symptoms appear within 2–3 days following the last drink and may last 3–5 days
- Nausea or vomiting
- Anxiety
- Depressed mood or irritability
- Malaise or weakness
- Autonomic hyperactivity
- Tachycardia
- Diaphoresis
- Elevated blood pressure
- Orthostatic hypotension
- Slight tremors (of hands, tongue, and eyelids) at rest, gross and irregular tremors during activities
- Sense of agitation and inner shakiness
- Insomnia with nightmares of seemingly real events
- Transitory hallucinations

- Alcoholic hallucinosis (peaks 24 hours after last drink): tremulousness plus vivid persecutory and auditory hallucinations, agitation, increased suicide and preassaultive potential
- Alcohol withdrawal syndrome (AWS) (peaks 24–48 hours after last drink): tremulousness plus delirium, generalized seizures, disorientation for time and place, visual hallucinations, agitation, panic level of anxiety
- "Rum fits" (peaks 24–48 hours after last drink): 2–6 generalized seizures, presence of AWS

Barbiturates and Similarly Acting Sedatives or Hypnotics Withdrawal (lorazepam, alprazolam, diazepam, chlordiazepoxide, chloral hydrate, methaqualone, secobarbital, phenobarbital, pentobarbital)

- Short-acting barbiturates and benzodiazapenes (BZDs) are associated with withdrawal symptoms within the first 24 hours after discontinuation
- Longer-acting barbiturates and BZDs are associated with withdrawal symptoms within 24–72 hours of discontinuation
- A deep sleep is followed by decreased respiration, coma, and sometimes death
- Nausea and vomiting
- Malaise or weakness
- Autonomic hyperactivity
- Tachycardia
- Diaphoresis
- Elevated blood pressure
- Anxiety
- Depression or irritability
- Orthostatic hypotension
- Coarse tremors of hands, tongue, eyelids
- Painful muscle contractions
- Seizures occurring for up to 2 weeks after withdrawal
- Status epilepticus (grand mal seizures succeeding each other with little or no intermission)
- Hallucinations

Opiod Withdrawal (heroin, morphine, hydromorphine, codeine, methadone)

- Opioids have the highest rate of withdrawal symptoms, at 90.8% (Schneider, Levenson & Schnoll, 2001)

- Because opioids are physically addictive, withdrawal is a threat
- Withdrawal symptoms may appear within a few hours after the last dose of a short-acting opioid such as heroin
- Most severe withdrawal occurs within 36–48 hours, with the symptoms gradually decreasing over 2 weeks
- With longer-acting opioids such as methadone, withdrawal symptoms may not appear for 2–3 days and may persist for 1–2 weeks
- During this stressful time the person craves the drug
- Withdrawal symptoms are influenza-like
- Dilated pupils
- Tearing
- Runny nose
- Piloerection
- Diaphoresis
- Diarrhea
- Fever
- Yawning
- Mild hypotension
- Tachycardia
- Insomnia
- Restlessness and irritability
- Muscle and joint pains
- Increased respiration
- Gastrointestinal symptoms
- Loss of appetite
- Babies born to addicted mothers are irritable, have high-pitched crying, increased respirations, fever, sneezing, yawning, and tremors

Cocaine withdrawal

- Symptoms may appear within 24 hours after use; peak in 2–4 days
- Anxiety, depression, and fatigue appear as the "postcoke blues," or cocaine abstinence syndrome
- Fatigue
- Psychomotor agitation

- Hypersomnia
- Irritability
- Depression (may persist for months)
- With crack cocaine, severe craving occurs within minutes to hours
- With crack cocaine, depression appears within 3–7 days and may persist for weeks
- Babies born to crack-addicted mothers are irritable and have tremors and muscle rigidity

Amphetamine withdrawal (dexadrine, methamphetamine)

- Depression
- Fatigue
- Disturbed sleep
- Dreaming
- Restlessness
- Disorientation

Polydrug Use

- Assess for polydrug use—most substance abusers use more than one drug, which complicates diagnosis and treatment and increases the hazards because of synergistic (potentiating) effects, additive effects, and paradoxical effects

General Hospital Clients

- Be alert to the possibility that clients being treated for physiologic illnesses may be substance abusers and in danger of withdrawal
- Symptoms that do not mesh with the condition under treatment may be symptoms of substance withdrawal
- Debilitation out of proportion to the problem for which the client is seeking treatment
- Physical findings that do not correlate with the client's chief complaint
- Unsteady gait, slurring of speech, dilated pupils, night sweats, chills, blackouts, tremors, skin tracks, abscesses, nasal septum perforation, and jaundice are all symptoms of substance abuse and indicate that the client will be withdrawing from the use of a chemical substance
- Weight loss, poor hygiene, and poor nutrition

- Symptoms of substance withdrawal described earlier in this section
- Ask specific questions about the client's use of alcohol and other substances

Chemically Dependent Health Care Providers

- Frequent absenteeism before and after days off; always working (in order to obtain supply)
- Irritability
- Abrupt mood changes; inappropriate affect
- Sloppy charting and client care
- Problems with drugs (missing drugs, frequent "wasting" of drugs, inaccurate records)
- Frequent errors in judgment
- Frequent disappearance from the assigned area
- Offering to give medication to clients
- Frequent night shift work
- Clients receiving medications from the health care provider complain of little or no pain relief

Interventions

General Interventions (Regardless of Substance)

- Substance abusers who are suicidal or acutely ill with symptoms of withdrawal are often treated in a medical-surgical unit of a general hospital or a detoxification unit. *Treatment of withdrawal is complicated and needs special attention by experienced and trained staff.*
- Attend to life-threatening physiologic symptoms first and monitor vital signs and respiratory and cardiovascular function. *Alcoholism or drug addiction issues are secondary to the need to keep the client safe and attend to physiologic needs. Clients in withdrawal are usually not amenable to "talking" therapies.*
- Decrease stimulation; provide a darkened quiet room. *A quiet unstimulating environment reduces the possibility of convulsions and decreases anxiety.*
- Point out reality to hallucinating clients and to those with illusions ("I know you are seeing things, and I know you are frightened. You are in the hospital and we are caring for you. There are no bugs or monsters here. You are safe and will feel better

soon.") *Provides comfort and support to the client and helps orient the client to reality.*

- Monitor fluid intake and output and provide adequate nutrition and fluids. *Many clients are dehydrated and have the potential for fluid volume deficit. Nutrition of substance-abusing clients is often poor.*

- Assess changes in level of consciousness. *Many substances and complications of withdrawal affect level of consciousness, particularly if the client is withdrawing from barbiturates.*

- Offer emotional support and encouragement to the client and the client's family. *Withdrawal is uncomfortable and stressful for the client and for family and friends who witness the client's distress.*

Withdrawal from Alcohol

- Monitor the client's fluid status and encourage up to 3000 ml/day if no evidence exists to contraindicate this (fluids may be administered intravenously). *Although some clients are overhydrated, many are dehydrated or have the potential for developing a fluid volume deficit.*

- Administer magnesium sulfate. *Administering magnesium sulfate decreases muscular irritability caused by low magnesium levels and prevents seizures.*

- Administer vitamins, especially thiamine (vitamin B1). *Alcohol interferes with the absorption of B vitamins.*

- Administer BZDs such as diazepam (may be given IV) or chlordiazepoxide, and phenytoin. *These medications help prevent AWS.*

- If client is prescribed disulfiram (Antabuse, an agonist medication), inform the client orally and in writing not to use alcohol in any form, including alcohol-based cough syrups, cold remedies, or mouthwashes. *Disulfiram interferes with the metabolism of acetaldehyde. As a result, acetaldehyde—which is highly toxic—accumulates if alcohol is consumed. If the client uses alcohol, a powerful disulfiram reaction may occur and last for up to 2 weeks. Reaction symptoms include nausea, vomiting, flushing, dizziness, tachycardia, and hypotension (which leads to shock and may be fatal).*

- Administer naltrexone. *Initially developed as a treatment for heroin abuse, this drug also blocks the craving for alcohol and the pleasure derived from drinking it. Because it does not make the alcoholic sick, it is a less punitive pharmacologic treatment than disulfiram.*

Withdrawal from Opioids

- Look for symptoms of opioid withdrawal 1–3 days after client is stabilized on methadone. *Methadone is used to stabilize symptoms and to treat opioid addiction.*
- Administer clonidine until withdrawal symptoms are alleviated (up to 14 days). *Clonidine blocks withdrawal symptoms, making the detoxification process less painful and more rapid than with methadone alone.*

Withdrawal from Cocaine

- Many hospitals use a diazepam protocol. *Diazepam protocols vary from PRN administration to four-day protocols that may include oral, IM or IV administration. Diazepam protocols depend on the client's symptoms and agency protocols. Some hospitals may not use a diazepam protocol.*
- Another protocol involves imipramine hydrochloride or other tricyclic antidepressants for several weeks after detoxification. *Depression may be severe and require treatment.*
- Administer beta-adrenergic blockers (such as propranolol). *Propranolol counteracts the tachycardia and hypertension that accompany acute intoxication.*
- Monitor vital signs, especially blood pressure.

Withdrawal from Amphetamines

- Administer medications such as chlorpromazine and diazepam. *Chlorpromazine combats the physiologic effects of amphetamines. Diazepam decreases tachycardia and the chance of convulsions.*

General Hospital Client

- Alert primary health care provider to the possibility of substance withdrawal. *It will be important for the primary care provider to institute treatment for withdrawal and to alter the plan of care based on this new information.*
- Suggest appropriate laboratory studies (such as liver function tests). *Laboratory studies will determine physiologic effects of substance abuse that may interfere with the client's treatment for the condition for which the client is hospitalized.*

- Encourage the client to seek treatment for substance abuse. *Recognizes substance abuse as a medical condition that requires intervention.*

Chemically Dependent Health Care Providers

- Be alert to behavior that suggests a problem. *Health care workers experience stress every day and have easy access to drugs; therefore, it can be an easy leap to self-medicate.*

- Attempt to talk with the coworker and encourage the coworker to seek help before documenting and reporting such behavior to a supervisor. *It is best if the individual is the person to acknowledge the problem and seek help for it.*

- If necessary, report the suspected behavior to a supervisor. *Shielding a health care provider, whatever the professional discipline, puts clients, the health care provider, and the profession at risk. It also violates professional practice, the code of ethics, and the law in many states.*

Communicating with a Substance-Using Client in Withdrawal

Client: "I feel so terrible. My muscles are twitching, I feel like I'm going to throw up, I'm dizzy and weak, and my heart is pounding. I'm so sorry I'm such a burden to you."

Nurse: "I'm going to take your blood pressure and your other vital signs now. We'll keep on top of your physical symptoms to keep you safe and take steps to make sure that you're more comfortable." *Rationale: This interaction treats the event as an illness in which there are physical consequences to one's behavior. It also reassures the client that the staff has the client's safety and comfort needs in mind.*	**Nurse:** "I'm going to take care of your physical needs right now, and then give you a little time to yourself. We'll talk later when you're better able to concentrate." *Rationale: An intoxicated client who is withdrawing is not able to benefit from a detailed discussion. This gives the client time to feel better once physical needs are attended to.*

SUBSTANCE-USING CLIENT: IN RECOVERY

Substance abuse is a chronic disease, often with remissions and exacerbations. While the outcome of total and permanent abstinence may be achievable for some clients with some abuse disorders, for others it may be an unattainable goal. Progress and relapse depend on the individual.

Assessment Cues

- Assess for symptoms of substance abuse
- Assess for symptoms leading to relapse:
  1. Fatigue and feelings of physical illness
  2. Rationalizing—making excuses for not doing what the person does not want to do, or for doing what the person knows he or she should not do
  3. Feeling impatient that things are not happening fast enough, or that others are not doing what they should do
  4. Arguing about small things; always wanting to be right
  5. Depression and negative feelings and thinking
  6. Frustration that everything is not the way the client wants it to be
  7. Self-pity (Why do these things happen to me? Nobody appreciates what I do for them.)
  8. Cockiness (I've got this problem licked, I have nothing to fear from drugs [booze])
  9. Complacency when things are going well (more relapses seem to occur when things are going well than when things are going badly)
  10. Expecting too much from others; expecting others to change their lifestyle because the client has
  11. Letting up on disciplines—such as prayer, meditation, daily inventory, 12-step meeting attendance—because of boredom with the recovery process or complacency
  12. Using mood-altering chemicals
  13. Setting goals that one cannot reach with normal efforts
  14. Forgetting gratitude for how much better life is now
  15. Acting as if "it can't happen to me"
  16. Feeling omnipotent, as if one has all the answers, and ignoring suggestions or advice from others

Interventions

- Intervention can occur as soon as the problem is identified. Educate family and friends on how to carry out a group intervention using the steps identified below. *Group intervention (confrontation) breaks through the client's denial.*

1. Presentation of facts: You had slurred speech and didn't even respond when I told you that I had to have surgery. You missed work for three days. You have alcohol on your breath (or needle marks on your arm). You haven't made your daughter's dinner all week and you forgot to pick her up from school. I found an empty bottle of vodka in your suitcase and water bottles filled with vodka instead of water in the refrigerator.

2. Consequences: Either you enter a treatment program now, or I will move out with the kids. Either you get help now, or you will have to leave your job. Either you get help now, or we'll find someone else to replace you on this project.

- Recovering clients may be treated in specialty hospital units specifically for the treatment of substance abuse, in residential rehabilitation facilities, in extended care facilities, and in community based programs. *The type of treatment program depends on several factors—the client's needs, availability, insurance, etc.*

- Refer client to self-help groups. *Support and self-help groups help clients feel better about themselves, direct them toward acquiring new behaviors, demonstrate that hope and recovery are possible, and provide new friends.*

  1. Support client in a spiritual fellowship program such as Alcoholics Anonymous (AA) and Narcotics Anonymous (NA) that focuses on abstinence as essential to recovery. *These are successful self-help groups in which people learn to change negative attitudes and behaviors into positive ones.*

  2. Support clients who reject a spiritual fellowship in programs such as Rational Recovery or Women for Sobriety, which inspire independence and suggest that until now the client has simply not chosen to stop the addiction. *Provides an alternative for clients who reject reliance on a higher power.*

- Help the individual to anticipate, and thus avoid, relapse by identifying situations of high risk that increase stress. *If the person can identify high-risk situations early, the individual can move to reduce stress.*

- Discuss with the client ways to alter destructive habits and the development of alternative coping strategies. *Identify destructive habits and develop new coping strategies that work to give clients confidence and will help to avoid relapse.*

- Encourage client to discover new interests. *Developing new interests provides other coping strategies.*

- Encourage the client in lifestyle changes—avoiding friends who are substance abusers or places or situations in which they used to take drugs or alcohol. *The mere sight or smell of paraphernalia or the desired substance is often enough to trigger a relapse. Old ties must be broken.*

- Set up a contract with the client, e.g., the client may agree to contact the nurse or an AA/NA sponsor when feeling the urge to drink or do drugs. *Developing a contract recognizes that relapse is always a threat. The agreement represents new behaviors necessary for a lifestyle change.*

- Provide psychoeducation by nurses, other experts, and recovered substance abusers who use culturally sensitive and relevant educational materials. *Knowledge and awareness may be useful in decreasing self-destructive behavior.*

Communicating with a Substance-Abusing Client in Recovery

Client: "I don't need to spend a lot of time talking to you about this stuff. I'm not going to take coke again, and you can bet on that."

Nurse: "I hear that you have no intentions to use cocaine again, and that's good. I also want to make sure that you have every support available to you when your resolve gets shaky." *Rationale: This interaction provides direction around the eventual difficulties that face everyone dependent on a substance—temptation and relapse.*	**Nurse:** "We don't have to do a lot of talking, but you have to make the changes in what you do and who you do it with." *Rationale: A clear statement about the client's responsibility for his own behavior and the necessary changes that need to be made interferes with urges to shift blame.*

SUICIDAL CLIENT

A suicidal client, whether child, adolescent, adult, or elder, has purposeful self-destructive thoughts, plans, or actions.

Assessment Cues

- Assess lethality by directly asking whether the client intends suicide. Questions include ideas or thoughts about suicide as well as any planning that may have taken place

- Determine whether the client has access to the method planned (such as access to pills, gun, rope, chemicals)
- Does not plan to be present for a near-future event that would normally be attended
- Giving away valued or cherished possessions
- Assess clients who are actively depressed—although clients diagnosed some time ago may generate the ability for self-harm once treatment begins to energize vegetative symptoms
- Lethality may become an option when a client perceives a rejection or an additional stressor (staff change, discharge, holiday, anniversary, promotion)
- Discuss the meaning of vague statements that could be construed as declaring self-harm (e.g., My mother won't have to worry about me anymore.)
- Components of a complete lethality assessment include: suicidal thoughts, plan, or attempts; prior self-destructive violence; concurrent chronic or severe acute medical problem; prior medication-resistant depression; social withdrawal; and decline in work productivity
- The risk for suicide is reduced somewhat, although not eliminated, when the client reports a decrease in suicidal thoughts and impulses and commits no acts of self-violence

Interventions

- Encourage clients to seek contact with a clinician when bothered by suicidal thoughts or impulses. *Discussion of these thoughts and impulses may be sufficient to diminish them and prevent a suicidal crisis from occurring. Do not reinforce suicidal ruminations by discussing them in detail.*
- Severely depressed and/or suicidal clients require inpatient treatment to ensure their safety. *The inpatient environment can be controlled and the client's urges managed with specialized staff in attendance. Suicidal clients need to know that the environment is safe for them. Reassure them by removing sharp objects, razors, breakable glass items, mirrors, matches, and straps or belts and explain why these objects are being removed. Monitor the use of scissors, razors, and other potential weapons.*
- Teach and reinforce alternative coping skills, such as substituting talking about problems instead of acting on an impulse because of a problem. *Clients need to have an array of*

competent coping choices so that suicide is not the only available response to a problem.

- Establish a behavioral contract where contingencies are listed and the client agrees to not harm self. *Safety contracts have been helpful to clients when resisting self-destructive urges, as a concrete reminder of the need for personal fortitude and outside assistance.*

- Discuss and alter the client's negative self-, world-, and future-view. *Talk about what negative thoughts the client has about himself and provide a list of neutral or positive statements to substitute for the negative.*

- Promote the client's identification of resources that can be helpful if suicidal thoughts return following discharge. *Reinforce how help is available from a variety of sources when the client's coping is insufficient.*

Communicating with a Suicidal Client

Client: "I would never want to be a burden to my wife."

Nurse: "Have you had thoughts about killing yourself so that you wouldn't be a burden?" *Rationale: Directly questioning and clarifying a communication that could indicate lethality.*	**Nurse: "Tell me what you would be doing that could be considered a burden."** *Rationale: Determining the client's definition of a burden and initiating neutral or positive statements to counter a negative self-view.*

SUSPICIOUS CLIENT

Suspiciousness is a way of thinking that reflects an attitude of doubt about the trustworthiness of objects or people. The suspicious person is usually preoccupied with being maneuvered, tricked, or framed.

Assessment Cues

- Believe that others plot against them or attempt to use or deceive them
- Talks about disloyal friends, coworkers, family members and staff members

- Are surprised by and mistrustful of loyalty shown to them
- May refuse to answer questions with the rationale "This is no one's business"
- Interprets behavior of others as premeditated
- Is overly concerned with hidden motives and special meanings, e.g., a birthday gift may be a trick to create an obligation
- Holds grudges and is unwilling to forgive
- Reports anger and disappointment at the actions of others
- Argumentative
- Tends to be hypervigilant—a far more attentive and acute observer than the ordinary person
- Suspicion of spousal or partner infidelity is a theme
- Hostile, stubborn sarcasm may predominate
- Is guarded and secretive
- Has a restricted affect and lack of spontaneity
- Tends to affiliate with special interest groups or cults with similar beliefs that reinforce the person's interpretations of reality—quasipolitical groups, esoteric religions, cults, or quasiscientific organizations

Interventions

- Respect the client's personal space, privacy, and preferences as much as is reasonable. *Predictable environments (schedules, consistent caregivers, etc.) decrease anxiety and foster trust.*
- Provide the client with a daily schedule of activities and inform the client of changes. *Activity schedules will diminish anxiety about social interactions and may help ensure the client's participation.*
- Use an objective, matter-of-fact approach. *The client will be able to identify the nurse as a reliable person who gives respect without argument.*
- Use concrete, specific words rather than global abstractions. *This will keep the intended message clear and limit the possibility of misinterpretation.*
- Respond to suspicious ideas by focusing on feelings ("It must be distressing . . .", "You see him as vindictive . . .") *Communicates empathy.*
- Avoid lengthy sessions with the client. Instead, conduct brief one-to-one sessions daily. *Shortened sessions decrease fear and anxiety.*

- Gradually introduce the client to group situations. *The presence of many people may be overwhelming. Allow the client to adjust to group situations gradually.*
- Help the client identify adaptive diversionary measures (e.g., leisure, recreation) in one-to-one sessions and groups. *Adaptive diversionary measures may reduce the client's focus on mistrust by occupying the client. Participation in groups may increase the client's support system.*
- Use role playing to help the client identify feelings, thoughts, and responses brought on by stressful situations. *Rehearsing social behaviors in a safe environment provides immediate feedback and time for altering responses.*
- Encourage the client to evaluate how client behaviors led to the current crisis. *This strategy points out the cause-and-effect aspects of interactions.*

Communicating with the Suspicious Client

Client: **"What did you mean by that remark? People are always making fun of me."**

Nurse: **"That remark was not meant for you, Jerry. It was directed toward everyone in the group."** *Rationale: This response provides a simple explanation without being argumentative or overly detailed in explanation. It also reinforces reality for the client.*	Nurse: **"You feel others are laughing at you."** *Rationale: Encourages the client to verbalize feelings of mistrust. When stated in a nonjudgmental manner by the nurse who maintains appropriate eye contact, this is a behavior that promotes trust.*

EVALUATION AND DOCUMENTATION

Evaluating is the last of the six standards of the nursing process. Care is an ongoing occurrence; evaluation is also continuous. It appraises nursing interventions, the impact of care on the client, and the client's outcomes. The evaluation of the care we have given to clients must compare the outcomes established for the problem areas to how the client is progressing towards more independent functioning in the identified area. The evaluation stage of the nursing process is an opportunity to examine not only the client's circumstances, but our own effectiveness as nurses. Were the outcomes, plans, and interventions appropriate? How could the nursing process have been enhanced for this client?

Measuring this evaluation takes place in a number of ways.

- Develop a mechanism, formal or informal, to determine the client's level of satisfaction with the care received.
- Determine the treatment's cost:benefit ratio.
- Document interventions, client responses to care, and alterations in plan and interventions in sufficient quantity, with necessary quality.
- Make the comparison between the plan of care and the outcomes.
- Make ongoing adjustments to diagnosis, plan of care, interventions, and outcomes.
- Determine whether consistency was maintained in the way care was managed.

CHARTING GUIDELINES

The client's record is a source of interdisciplinary communication. It is a legal document logging what has been done, offering information contributing to decision-making about what could be done, and keeping track of the ongoing relationship between the client and health care providers. Documentation is more than test results, diagnostic impressions, historical data, and current interactions. It shapes the client's care and can alter events.

Documentation in a client's record must contain a number of features.

- Handwritten documents must be legible. Signature and title must also be legible.
- All documentation must use proper and explicit grammar so that misunderstandings and garbled communications are minimized.
- Electronic documents usually cannot be altered once they are entered and verified. Each entry must reflect exactly what the writer intends, as addendums are the only means of correction.
- Confidentiality of all client health information according to the Health Information Portability and Accountability Act (HIPAA) must be assured.
- There is an explicit plan of care, including which discipline is responsible and accountable for which methods of intervention.

- Lethality-related information must be clearly articulated, including any change in behavior, gifting treasured items, etc.
- The client's progress towards goals is documented.
- Information from auxiliary sources (such as family, significant others, other health care providers, neighbors, agencies, schools, employers, community, and authorities) is documented and attributed to that source.
- Every change to care that is made—as well as a decision not to make a change—along with a rationale, is documented so that the clinician's thinking is apparent from the record.
- Documentation includes the nursing care given, communications held, information shared, procedures performed, and any other data about the client's care useful to the interdisciplinary treatment team.
- Communication in the record of the client's response to the nursing care given.
- Patterns of client response and interaction are important features of documented information.
- Charting in a particular style may be used to cover all critical areas of nursing care:
  1. SOAP notes for Subjective (what the client is saying), Objective (the clinician's perspective), Assessment (judgment made from data the clinician collected), Plan (an organized intervention strategy in response to the assessment)
  2. IOAP notes for Input (what the nurse did for or with the client), Output (how the client responded to that interaction), Assessment (judgment made from data the clinician collected), Plan (an organized intervention strategy in response to the assessment)

PRACTICE BASED ON RESEARCH

Nursing is a science based on fact. We need facts to direct our decision-making and enhance our care. These facts have been established as a result of careful examination of client care. The most meaningful examination of a care situation is one where the information is:

- Unbiased
- Can be used with a majority of people who have similar problems
- Is not likely to have happened just as a matter of luck or chance.

This examination is called research. The Code for Federal Research (CFR) governing research activities in the Unites States, 45 CFR 46, defines research as "a systematic investigation, including research development, testing, and evaluation, designed to develop or contribute to generalizable knowledge."

Assuring Bias-Free Research

An important research priority is to assure that it is free of bias. In research, bias is defined as:

- Following a procedure that changes or alters the results of the study—often in a way that suits the needs of the researcher—although bias can also happen accidentally or inadvertently.

- Intentional bias includes situations where the researcher evaluates two alternative ways of performing an intervention, but favors one approach over another. Staff may deliver the preferred intervention with more diligence and enthusiasm than with the alternative intervention. This can produce results that seem to indicate the favored intervention is superior, yet the outcome instead may have been produced by a difference in enthusiasm on the part of the researcher.

- A subtle form of bias can occur if two interventions are delivered to nonequivalent groups of clients. This could occur when the researcher favors one intervention over the other and selects clients who are less ill or who are more likely to improve from that favored intervention. The resulting superior outcomes for the favored intervention will reflect a bias in sampling rather than an actual outcome difference resulting from the intervention.

- Unintentional bias can occur in research where the researcher persists in performing different statistical analyses until finally a statistically significant result is generated. In this case, the result is a function of the random chance that given a large enough number of analyses, one or two will always generate significant findings. This does not reflect any actually significant study findings.

You can see that bias can take many forms. It is an important research responsibility to be vigilant in detecting possibilities for bias and establishing research procedures that eliminate, or greatly minimize, bias.

Types of Research

Nursing professionals perform and use research employing a wide variety of techniques. Types of research include:

- Quantitative research studies look statistically (using quantities or numbers) at a nursing intervention. These studies can be fully experimental research designs which permit the researcher to evaluate the effectiveness of that intervention as compared to others, or to a placebo procedure.
- Qualitative research explores the qualities of a human experience. An example of this type of research is a study in which the researcher interviews or surveys clients about their perceptions and opinions of the treatment they have received.
- Retrospective review research studies are those in which the researcher reviews charts and other documentation of client care retrospectively, looking for patterns in the documented results of that treatment which bear on treatment effectiveness.

Increasingly, nursing research seeks to integrate these and other methodological approaches to produce research findings that are precise, informative, and illustrative.

Additional Priorities in Research

When nursing research is conducted, there are additional priorities above and beyond the soundness or completeness of the study design. These include protection of research participants, the ethics of the study, and seeking informed consent from research participants. Adherence to federal and local regulations is required. It is also expected that researchers will analyze their research data in an unbiased, competent, and objective fashion as well as share and communicate their research findings clearly and openly.

An example of research that is generalizable, as stated in the CFR definition of research, would be a study completed on people diagnosed as having schizophrenia. Once the study results are shared in the literature or through professional presentations, nurses could incorporate the research findings into their practices. The research results and conclusions could be generalized and applied to a different group of people with schizophrenia than the ones studied.

Basing Practice on Research

How you base your nursing practice activities on research involves incorporating an intervention that has been studied scientifically and proves to be successful into your repertoire. For example, hundreds of HIV-positive client cases were reviewed to determine why treatment regimens were discontinued when they were working "well," meaning test results were improving. Research showed that clients who have symptoms of depression miss appointments and do not adhere to medication regimens. Depression was also found to increase the intensity of HIV symptoms and lower the quality of life for the client. If your practice was based on research evidence, you would incorporate a depression screening interview and interventions to relieve the symptoms of depression to stem the flow of nonadherence to life-saving assistance.

Resources for your professional need–incorporating research findings into practice-abound. Advanced practice nurses, professional organizations, Web-based resources for evidence-based nursing, agencies (such as the Agency for Healthcare Research and Quality, AHRQ), government databases (such as the National Guidelines Clearinghouse), and your facility's own resources will help you perform this outstanding nursing function.

BIBLIOGRAPHY

Aguilera, D.C. (1998). *Crisis intervention: Theory and methodology*. St. Louis, MO: Mosby.

American Nurses Association (2000). *Scope and standards of psychiatric-mental health nursing practice*. Washington, DC: American Psychiatric Nurses Association.

American Nurses Association (2001). *Code of ethics for nurses*. Washington, DC: Author.

American Psychiatric Association, (2000). *Diagnostic and statistical manual of mental disorders* (4th ed., Text Revision), Washington, DC: Author

American Psychiatric Nurses Association. (2000). *Position statement on the use of seclusion and restraint*. Retrieved January 20, 2003, from the World Wide Web, *www.apna.org*.

Barnsteiner, J. & Prevost, S. (2002). How to implement evidence-based practice: Some tried and true pointers. *Reflections on Nursing Leadership, 28*, 18–21.

CDC, 1988. Perspectives in disease prevention and health promotion update: Universal precautions for prevention of transmission of human immunodeficiency virus, hepatitis B virus, and other bloodborne pathogens in health-care settings. *www.cdc.gov/wonder/prevguid*.

Fontaine, K.L. (2000). *Healing Practices: Alternative Therapies for Nursing*. Upper Saddle River, NJ: Prentice Hall.

Fontaine, K.L. & Fletcher, J.S. (2003). *Mental Health Nursing*. (5th ed.). Upper Saddle River, NJ: Prentice Hall.

Hart, L.A. (2000). Psychosocial benefits of animal companionship. In A.H. Fine (ed.), *Handbook on animal-assisted therapy* (pp. 59–78). San Diego, CA: Academic Press.

Holzemer, W.L. (2002). HIV and AIDS: The symptom experience. *American Journal of Nursing, 102*, 48–52.

Johnson, M., Maas, M., & Moorhead, S. (2000). *Nursing outcomes classification (NOC)* (second ed.). St. Louis, MO: Mosby.

Kapp, D.A. (2000). *The burden of sympathy: How families cope with mental illness*. London: Oxford University Press.

Kessler, R.C., Walters, E.E., & Forthofer, M.S. (2001). The use of complementary and alternative therapies to treat anxiety and depression in the United States. *American Journal of Psychiatry, 158*(2), 289–294.

Kneisl, C.R., Wilson, H., and Trigoboff, E. (2004). *Contemporary Psychiatric–Mental Health Nursing.* Upper Saddle River, NJ: Prentice Hall.

Lieck, D.J. & Bertram, J.E. (2002). Drug accountability at the investigative site. *Applied Clinical Trials, 11*, 36–44.

Marshall, T.B., & Solomon, P. (2000). Releasing information to families of persons with severe mental illness: A survey of NAMI members. *Psychiatric Services, 51*(8), 1006–1011.

McCloskey, J., & Bulechek, G.M. (2000). *Nursing interventions classification (NIC)* (3rd ed.). St. Louis, MO: Mosby.

Mead, S., & Copeland, M.E. (2000). What recovery means to us: Consumers' perspectives. *Community Mental Health Journal, 36*(3), 315–328.

National Institutes of Health (2001). Institution of universal precautions. NIH Clinical Center Nursing Department. *www.cc.nih. gov/nursing/univer.html.*

North American Nursing Diagnosis Association (2003). *Nursing diagnoses, definitions and classifications, 2003–2004.* Philadelphia: Author.

Occupational Safety and Health Administration (2000). *Guidelines for workplace violence prevention programs for health care and social service workers.* Washington, DC: U.S. Department of Labor.

Ratey, J.J. (2001). *A user's guide to the brain.* New York: Pantheon Books.

Roberts, A.R. (2000). *Crisis intervention handbook: Assessment, treatment, and research.* (2nd ed.). New York: Oxford University Press.

Rosenstein, A.H. (2002). Original research: Nurse–physician relationships' impact on nursing satisfaction and retention. *American Journal of Nursing, 102*, 26–34.

Schneider, R.K., Levenson, J.L., & Schnoll, S.H. (2001). Update in addiction medicine. *Annals of Internal Medicine, 134*, 387–395.

Teschinsky, U. (2000). Living with schizophrenia: The family illness experience. *Issues in Mental Health Nursing, 21*(4), 387–396.

Whittemore, R. & Grey, M. (2002). The systematic development of nursing interventions. *Journal of Nursing Scholarship, 34*, 115–120.

Wuerker, A.K. (2000). The family and schizophrenia. *Issues in Mental Health Nursing*, 21(1), 127–141.

Yalom, I.D. (1995). *The theory and practice of group psychotherapy.* (4th ed.). New York: Basic Books.

Test, M.A., & Stein, L.I. (2000) Practical guidelines for the community treatment of markedly impaired patients. *Community Mental Health Journal,* 36(1), 47–60.

Wilson, B.A., Shannon, M.T., & Stang, C.L. (2003) *Nurse's drug guide 2003.* Upper Saddle River, NJ: Prentice Hall.

INDEX

A

abdominal pain, lithium and, 135
abuse. *See also* substance abuse
  DSM codes related to, 25
  NOC assessment of, 77–78
  protection from, 84
  rape-trauma treatment, 83
abusive behavior, NOC assessment of, 75
Activities of Daily Living (ADLs), 94–95
activity/exercise management, 80
activity therapy, 80
  groups, 101
acupressure, 110–111
acupuncture, 110–111
Addison's disease, weight loss and, 61
adjustment disorders, DSM codes for, 24
advance directives, psychiatric, 45
adynamic ileus, chlorpromazine and, 130
aggression
  aggressive responses and, 86
  anger and, 82, 157–158
  clinical applications for, 151–155
  NOC assessment of control, 75
  sexual, clinical applications for, 155–156
agitation. *See also* nervousness
  buproprion and, 125
  olanzapine and, 139
agranulocytosis, chlorpromazine and, 130
AIDS/HIV
  depression and, 208–209
  DSM codes for dementia related to, 12
  universal precautions for, 46–47
AIMS (Abnormal Involuntary Movement Scale), 8
alcohol
  olanzapine and, 140
  trazodone and, 144
  valproic acid and, 147
alcoholism. *See also* substance abuse
  CAGE diagnostic for, 7–8
  DSM codes for disorders related to, 13

herbal medicine and, 113
trazodone for, 142–145
withdrawal, assessment of, 190–191
withdrawal, interventions for, 195–196
alertness, aromatherapy and, 112. *See also* drowsiness
alien control, delusions of, 56
alprazolam, 119–121
  nefazadone and, 138
alternative therapies, 110–116
  acupuncture, 110–111
  animal-assisted, 111
  aromatherapy, 111–112
  ayurveda, 112
  chiropractic, 112–113
  curanderismo, 113
  herbal medicine, 113–114
  hypnotherapy and guided imagery, 114
  massage, 114
  meditation, 114–115
  Native American, 115
  prayer, 115
  T'ai Chi, 115–116
  therapeutic touch, 116
  traditional Chinese medicine, 112
  yoga, 116
Alzheimer's disease. *See also* dementia
  DSM codes for, 11
  PET scans in, 6
American Nurses' Association (ANA)
  Code of Ethics for Nurses, 36
  standards of practice, 3–5
Amitril, 121–124
amitriptyline, 121–124
amnestic disorders, DSM codes for, 12. *See also* memory
amphetamines. *See also* substance abuse
  DSM codes for disorders related to, 13–14
  psychosis related to, 60
  withdrawal, assessment of, 193
  withdrawal, interventions for, 196